Proven Solutions for Improving Health and Lowering Health Care Costs

Proven Solutions for Improving Health and Lowering Health Care Costs

by

C. Carl Pegels
School of Management
University at Buffalo

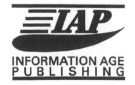

INFORMATION AGE
PUBLISHING

80 Mason Street
Greenwich, Connecticut 06830

Library of Congress Cataloging-in-Publication Data

Pegels, C. Carl.
  Proven solutions for improving health and lowering health care costs /
C. Carl Pegels.
      p. cm. – (The proven solutions series)
Includes bibliographical references.
  ISBN 1-59311-000-6 (pbk) – ISBN 1-59311-001-4 (hc)
  1. Health services administration. I. Title. II. Series.
  RA971.P395 2003
  362.1'068–dc21

                                    2003000191

Printed in the United States of America

CONTENTS

PREFACE

Health Science research, especially health research outcomes with direct implications for health improvement, are quickly disseminated by the popular press. The same cannot be said for scientific health management research and scientific general management research.

Scientific research is published in academic research journals which are typically only read by other scientific management researchers. Some of these research results may eventually find their way into management textbooks, but these textbooks generally only provide exposure to management students and their professors. The potential immediate beneficiaries of the scientific management research results, the professional health system managers, seldom are exposed to this research.

The barrier that stands in the way of scientific management research and the professional health systems manager is the language used to publish the research. Scientific research utilizes extensive and sophisticated statistical tools with which the professional health systems manager is not familiar, and as a result does not understand. Because of this barrier the publishers of scientific management journals do not promote their journals to professional health systems managers.

Another barrier standing in the way of the dissemination of scientific management research is the abundance of popular management literature written by the so-called management gurus. There is a veritable flood of books on the market providing professional managers with enough read-

Proven Solutions for Improving Health and Lowering Health Care Costs, pages vii–10.
Copyright © 2003 by Information Age Publishing, Inc.
All rights of reproduction in any form reserved.
ISBN: 1-59311-000-6 (paper), 1-59311-001-4 (cloth)

ing material to keep their free time well occupied. There is now even a top ten list of business books.

The problem with the popular management literature is that most of it is based on the writer's opinion, and has seldom been scientifically tested. The published material is often referred to as armchair wisdom. Even if the material is based on a successful case study, the case study typically consists of a sample of one, and is seldom generalizable to other situations or organizations.

Proven Solutions for Improving Health and Lowering Health Care Costs is a collection of well over 100 descriptions of scientific management studies in the field of health care or relevant to health care. Each one of the scientific studies is presented in readable and understandable form for individuals who probably have not had the statistical and scientific education and training to fully understand the underlying scientific studies.

We can also view each of the well over 100 descriptions as translations of scientific management research, translated so the results can be quickly grasped and understood by the non-scientific reader. In other words the busy health systems manager does not need to waste his or her time trying to understand the scientific article. By reading the translations he or she can at a quick grasp of the scientific results of all the included scientific studies.

The book is significantly different from the popular management literature which is based on "arm-chair" management experts who use current facts or at best use anecdotal references to publicize their ideas.

Although the book is targeted for the health systems manager/administrator it can also be used as a supplementary reader in such courses as Health Administration, Nursing Administration, Health Policy, Health Economics, Health Marketing, Health Care Finance, Informatics in Health Care; etc.

Acknowledgments: I would like to thank all the students who contributed to the development of this book through the contribution of research translation drafts of individual published research papers. Special thanks goes to Paula Frazier who provided several of such contributions. Others who contributed and deserve special thanks are Allison Allport, Daniel Avoso, Michelle Arteaga, Kira Baranska, Debbie Buckley, Daniel Butzer, Thomas DiScipio, Robert Giardini, Michelle Gliss, Susan Hanson, Rosemary Holmberg, Susan Judd, Jennifer Kozinski, Lora Melchow, Eileen Nahigian, Jennifer Schuleford, Ebrahim Randeree, and John Wood.

I also want to express my thanks to Valerie Limpert for an outstanding job of typing and proofreading several versions of the manuscript, and to my wife, Patricia, for providing moral support during the preparation of this book.

C. Carl Pegels

CHAPTER 1

HIGHLIGHTS OF RESEARCH RESULTS

The purpose of this book is to convince administrators and providers of health care that scientific research has produced numerous tools, techniques, and approaches for managing health services that are most effective and most efficient. Convincing the managers and administrators of this fact is accomplished by presenting numerous easy-to-understand summaries of the research reported in the scientific research journals available at University and main city libraries.

The easy-to-understand summaries of the research reports can also be typified as research translations or interpretations. We have organized these research translations into 15 chapters covering such areas as Health Policy, Health Economics, Health Marketing, Health Cost Issues, Total Quality Management, Informatics, Human Resource Management, Managed Care, Clinical Issues, and others.

Below we will give brief descriptions of some of the more interesting studies largely based on their interest level to health system administrators and health care providers. The reports you will read below are based on scientific research, and not on anecdotal stories.

Much of the popular management literature in book stores, in the top 10 business books, and on managers' bookshelves are so-called managerial

Proven Solutions for Improving Health and Lowering Health Care Costs, pages 1–10.
Copyright © 2003 by Information Age Publishing, Inc.
All rights of reproduction in any form reserved.
ISBN: 1-59311-000-6 (paper), 1-59311-001-4 (cloth)

"wisdoms" which have no or little relationship to fact as determined by scientific empirical research. This book has been written to provide health and hospital administrators and health care providers with a collection of managerial facts which have been tested out scientifically.

In this chapter are about fifty of these scientifically-based managerial facts. In the remainder of the book each of about 113 of these scientific managerial facts are described in easy-to-understand detail. Each fact is referenced with a citation to the study which provided the specific scientific facts reported below.

1.1   HEALTH POLICY AND ITS IMPLICATIONS

Three studies are of particular interest in this chapter. The first is a study of deaths caused by radon gas. Although the country-wide death rate is relatively low, it still is an area where implementation of health policy can ameliorate the total annual death toll. Smoking causes about one-third of all the radon deaths in the U.S. Any reduction in smoking will of course have a concomitant impact on radon death rates. But smoking levels appear to be stabilizing and as a result not much reduction in radon death rates can be expected. The remaining two-thirds of radon death rates is from general exposure of naturally-generated radon levels in homes and other buildings. Control of radon exposure is therefore difficult unless every home and building in the country is inspected and if exposure to radon gases is present, then radon gas protective equipment needs to be installed. The cost of doing this is enormous and the researchers recommend a focus on those geographic areas where radon gas exposure is prominent and extensive.

The second study explores the effectiveness of clinical guidelines with a specific application to emergency room care. The researchers found that external application of guidelines is not very effective because the reasons behind the guidelines are not always well understood. However, in those cases where clinical guidelines are established with the participation of health care providers and clinicians the implemented guidelines were much more effective.

The third study looked at the problems of doing medical research where patient consent is required whenever data is used from patients' medical records. In one particular study it was found that a patient's consent was difficult to obtain even though the data used from the medical record would not be traceable back to the patient. As a result medical studies will be severely compromised and the results of these medical studies will not be as effective as they could be. The only explanation for the patient's refusal to participate could be their concern that the researcher or data recorder would be able to view their medical records.

1.2   HEALTH ECONOMICS

This chapter produced five studies of interest. The first study describes the results of an investigation to determine if collusion was used by health system employers in a regional area to set salary levels. The study was motivated by the fact that during nurse shortage periods salary levels generally would not budge. The results of the investigation revealed that collusion among employers was not present. The lower and firm salary levels were attributed to the fact that there was a lot of substitution in the nursing area. Licensed practical nurses could be substituted in many cases for registered nurses, and nurses' aids could be substituted for licensed practical nurses in some instances.

The second study addressed the issue of whether lower cost drugs are as cost-effective as higher-priced drugs. The focus was on the comparison of two antibiotics, one costing $247 and the other $295 per treatment. The researchers found that the high-cost antibiotic was more effective and more economically beneficial than the lower-priced drug.

The third study looked at internal development versus external hiring of employees. Which approach is more economical in the long run? The results show that internal development of current employees is more effective and economically beneficial than external hiring.

The fourth study explored whether care episodes in mental health care initiated by non-specialist physicians are as effective and as expensive as those initiated by non-physician providers. The research found that there was no difference between the two provider types in terms of costs or efficiency. However, the selection of type of provider by the client was affected by out-of-pocket costs by the client.

The fifth study looked at the cost of obesity. The researchers found that the cost of obesity in the U.S. amounts to about $70 billion per year. The three major cost components consist of cardiovascular problems amounting to about $30 billion per year, indirect costs of morbidity and mortality amounting to about $19 billion per year, and diabetes problems amounting to about $9 billion per year. The remaining $12 billion per year was caused by miscellaneous other diseases.

1.3   HEALTH CARE COSTS, EFFECTIVENESS, AND QUALITY ISSUES

The four studies of particular interest are summarized below. The first study provides an analysis of administrative costs in U.S. hospitals, much of it related to third party-related payment issues. The study's particular point of interest is the comparison with Canadian hospitals. In Canada, because of National Health Insurance, administrative costs in hospitals only amount to 9 percent of total costs. The comparable figure in U.S. hospitals is 25 percent of total hospital cost.

The second study describes a prediction model for hospital closures based on accounting ratios. The model is amazingly accurate and any hospital in precarious or even weak financial conditions may want to apply the model to evaluate its likelihood of survival.

The third study is a study of the effectiveness and costs of home-based care for terminally-ill patients. The study was based on Veterans Administration System patients. The study revealed that not only were patients cared for at home more economical to care for, but the quality of care as measured by patient satisfaction was significantly higher.

The fourth study evaluates the effects of occupational stress on the costs of health care. Not surprisingly, people suffering from occupational stress incurred higher health care costs. Some modification of the health care costs resulted from social support.

1.3 HEALTH MARKETING AND PROMOTION

In this chapter five studies are of particular interest. The first study shows the effectiveness of exercise to reduce occupational physical problems such as back aches. The study's purpose is to determine if physical exercise facilities provided by employers are effective to ameliorate the problems of occupation-induced physical problems. Although the benefits of physical exercise are unquestionable, the problem is the lack of interest in physical exercise by the majority of employees.

The second study shows that in advertising the quality of the ads is critical to their effectiveness. As a result it is suggested to devote considerable resources to ad design. Funds spent on ad design are much more effective than those same funds spent on ad exposure.

The third study focuses on personal solicitation for funds. The researchers found that the time and effort on preparing personal messages to each individual donor are most effective in producing positive and generous responses.

The fourth study revealed that chain pharmacies have considerably more bargaining power with mass purchasers such as health maintenance organizations. As a result individual pharmacies should be allowed to form cooperative type arrangements with other individual pharmacies to ensure them an opportunity for survival.

The fifth study revealed that rural hospitals will have serious difficulty to survive. Because of their smaller size rural hospitals cannot provide the same range of services provided by the larger urban hospitals. Younger families especially prefer to travel the longer distances to urban hospitals to ensure they receive the best possible care that is available.

1.5   TOTAL QUALITY MANAGEMENT IN HEALTH SYSTEMS

Three studies are of specific interest in this chapter. The first study shows that pay inequity can have negative effects on quality. This applies when senior management members pay themselves high salaries while attempting to keep the salaries of the remaining staff members as low as possible.

The second study shows that hospitals with positive corporate cultures will show better results from total quality management efforts. Positive corporate culture refers to ability by employers to handle change, successful use of team work by employees and empowered employees, among others. In other words developing a positive culture may well be a prerequisite for successful total quality management efforts.

The third study shows that successful applications of total quality management improve productivity and resultant profitability. In other words the dictum quality pays is found to be true if one is successful with a total quality management campaign. Be aware that not every total quality management campaign is successful.

1.6   CONTINUOUS QUALITY IMPROVEMENT IN HEALTH SYSTEMS

There are three studies of interest in this chapter. The first study reveals that the Malcolm Baldrige National Quality Assessment (MBNQA) method is a valid approach to improve quality and operational results. The MBNQA method is used by literally thousands of organizations annually to evaluate their operations. Organizations going through this rather time and resource consuming activity may feel assured that their time and effort is well spent.

The second study focused on the joint application of technology use and employee participation to improve quality and operational results. The researchers found that the joint application of the two approaches produced better results than the sum of each approach used individually.

The third study explored the effectiveness of diagnostic techniques preceding the performance of appendectomies in the United Kingdom. The study revealed that appendectomies could be reduced by one third if better diagnostic procedures were available.

1.7   OPERATIONS MANAGEMENT IN HEALTH SYSTEMS

In this chapter we cover two studies including one on nurse staffing levels and one on team performance. Nurse staffing levels in hospitals are almost universally based on patient load. The researchers studied this area and their research concluded that nurse staffing levels should be based both on patient loads and on the need levels of patients. Without considering patient need levels the workloads of nurses in hospitals can be significantly affected both in terms of overload and in terms of underutilization.

The second study looked at team performance and specifically at the performance of work teams. The question they posed was why there is so much variability in team performance. The researchers discovered that team performance is most effective and productive if team members are highly trained, have high seniority, and have high cohesion. Hence, presence of the three factors can be viewed as prerequisites for effective team performance.

1.8   INFORMATICS AND HEALTH CARE

Three studies are particularly significant in this chapter. The first study explores information systems in Health Maintenance Organizations (HMOs). The overall conclusion of the study is that HMO information systems are weak. Most systems have poor connectivity and continuity. There is little integration and as a result the systems are unable to provide necessary information especially of a clinical nature.

The second study explores how effective computer-generated reminders of the need for influenza immunizations are for seniors. The reminders are computer-generated and remind seniors to arrange an appointment for the immunization. The researchers found that the reminders significantly increased the participation rate by seniors in influenza immunizations.

The third study focuses on customer satisfaction with software packages. Numerous factors were evaluated by a large panel of software users. The researchers found that the three most critical influences on customer satisfaction with software packages were capability, usability, and performance.

1.9   HUMAN RESOURCE MANAGEMENT IN HEALTH SYSTEMS

This chapter contains five particular studies of interest to the Health Systems Manager. The first study focuses on absence behavior of employees and its relationship to absence standards in the work place. If an organiza-tion's culture looks benignly on absence behavior of employees, then the frequency of absences is greater than if the culture is judgmental of absen-teeism. Hence, it behooves management to create an atmosphere where unnecessary absence is not condoned.

The second study focuses on work environments in which employees thrive and are highly productive and effective. The researchers found that employees thrive in an environment of management commitment to the employees. An environment where management exercises tight control on its employees did not fare well in terms of employee performance. Also the researchers found that money is not a prime motivator but management commitment is.

The third study focuses on top management motivation. The research-ers explored the utilization of available cash flow by top managers. They found that top managers who utilized the available cash flow for business opportunities showed better long-term performance than managers who kept the available cash flow for just-in-case future situations

The fourth study is a gender study. The researchers explored the salary levels of men and women in salaried positions with the purpose of deter-mining if gender discrimination existed. They found that important salary factors were level of education, degree of experience, and employee-origi-nated restrictions, but not gender. Hence, in their study they did not find gender discrimination.

The fifth and final study questioned whether job satisfaction is related to intelligence. They found that job satisfaction is maximized if an individ-ual is matched to a job that requires that individual's level of intelligence. In other words people need a certain degree of challenge in their jobs. If the challenge is not there or is excessive, that individual's job satisfaction will be diminished.

1.10   ORGANIZATIONAL BEHAVIOR IN HEALTH SYSTEMS

Three studies of special interest are described below. The first study evalu-ates the effect of humor on three types of leadership behaviors. The researchers found that humor ameliorates the negative effects of transfor-mational leadership. However, humor had no effect on either contingent award leadership or on laissez-faire leadership behavior.

The second study looked at the effects of gender and gender-type behavior on leadership emergence in groups working together as a team on a project. The researchers found that gender had no effect on leader-ship emergence, but masculine behavior by either a man or a woman sig-nificantly affected leadership emergence.

The third study found that both trust and distrust are important and valuable in organizations. Trust is important in interpersonal relationships and information sharing. But distrust as reflected in control systems is also important to ensure that honesty prevails.

1.11   INSTITUTIONAL ISSUES IN HEALTH SYSTEMS

This chapter contains two studies of specific interest. The first study explores the skills required by an organization to be successful at alliance building. The researchers found that the most successful alliance builders were those organizations that had experimented with collaborative activities with other organizations in the past. Hence, learning is the key to be successful at alliance building.

The second study focuses on innovation by hospitals, and what factors cause a hospital to be more innovative than others. The researchers found that a high degree of innovation occurred in those hospitals which had many institutional links with other organizations.

1.12   MANAGERIAL ISSUES IN HEALTH SYSTEMS

This chapter had three studies of special interest. The first study explores focussing or specialization in health care institutions. The researchers found that not all hospitals have the luxury of focussing on special services. However, those hospitals which specialized in a limited number of services had higher operational efficiency, higher patient satisfaction, and higher staff satisfaction. These results are not surprising since specialization enables an organization to take advantage to quickly move down (or up) the learning curve.

The second study explores the successes and failures of entrepreneurial activities, both within firms and by outsiders. The researchers found that failure must be expected whenever an entrepreneurial activity is engaged in. Again experience in attempting numerous entrepreneurial activities is beneficial because the organization learns to be more selective and learns to avoid actions that lead to failure. For that reason the researchers recommend that organizations should analyze failures and learn from them in order to avoid future failures.

The third study looks at managerial decision making. The focus of the study was to determine if managers make satisficing versus optimizing decisions. The researchers found that managers will generally make satisficing decisions because they usually produce less conflict and as a result minimize stress on the managerial decision makers.

1.13 STRATEGIC MANAGEMENT IN HEALTH SYSTEMS

Three studies of special interest are described below. The first study explores whether cognitive (good) conflict or affective (dysfunctional) conflict produces better results. Not surprisingly the researchers found that cognitive conflict produced substantial better results than affective conflict.

The second study posed the question if hospital ownership conversions, from non-profit to for-profit and from for-profit to non-profit are beneficial to the survival of those organizations. The researchers found that ownership conversions of either type benefit those organizations by producing improved revenues and improved profit margins.

The third study posed a similar question as the one above. The question is if privatization improves productivity. The sample in this case encompassed more than just the hospital sector. It included any range of organizations which were privatized. The researchers found that privatization improves productivity especially if the chief executive officer is changed following the privatization.

1.14 MANAGED HEALTH CARE

There were two studies of special interest in this chapter. The first study explored if managed care and specifically a Health Maintenance Organization (HMO) influenced patients and providers to use strategies that will reduce cost. The researchers found that the cost control influences of the HMO had an impact on strategies used by both patient and provider. These strategies also were less costly. But the most interesting result of the study was that providers also adopted the same strategies for their fee-for-service patients and reduced the costs for their health care also.

The second study looked at why people use higher versus lower-premium health insurance. Although higher-premium health insurance provides broader coverage, the added premium cost does not always provide commensurate additional benefits. The researchers found that most of the higher premium plans were chosen by woman decision makers. Apparently women are willing to pay for the relatively smaller risk entailed in the lower premium health insurance plans.

1.15 CLINICAL HEALTH RESEARCH ISSUES

The last chapter has four studies of special interest. The first study covers the efficacy of neurology services for stroke patients. Stroke patients were either admitted to neurology services or non-neurology services in a given hospital over an extended time period. Stroke-in-evolution patients went generally directly to neurology services while other patients could be admitted to either service unit. The researchers found that neurology-services stroke patients generally made better progress and had lower mortality than stroke patients admitted to non-neurology services.

The second study covered the effect of guidelines on hypertensive patients. The researchers found that implementation of guidelines produced improvement in hypertension patients' ability to lower their blood pressure goals.

The third study covered self-management by nurses. The researchers studied two groups of nurses, one under self-management and the other supervised and directed by a supervisor. The study revealed that the self-managed group of nurses had significantly higher job satisfaction than the supervised group. However, there was no difference between the two groups in terms of effectiveness of services performed.

The fourth study focused on the effect of volume on knee replacement surgery in a hospital measured in terms of complications following surgery. The researchers found that there is a definite improvement in the quality of the surgery as volume increases, but the improvement does not increase in a linear fashion. Up to 80 knee replacement surgeries per year in a hospital produced a decided improvement as volume increased, but in hospitals which had in excess of 80 knee replacement surgeries per year, no improvement was found. Hence, the critical minimum number of knee replacements a hospital should be expected to perform amounted to 80 surgeries per year.

CHAPTER 2

HEALTH POLICY AND ITS IMPLICATIONS

This chapter will explore several health areas where federal and state health care policies have been of particular interest.

The first study addresses investor response to health care cost containment legislation. Federal policies to control health care costs have the potential to negatively affect the business prospects of for-profit organizations, and specifically for their ability to maintain their profitability. The premise of the study is that there will be no change in stock market performance of the affected firms if the investors in these firms anticipate the failure of the health care cost legislation. Two events were selected to evaluate the performance of a sample of 20 firms. The first event was the 1974 National Health Planning and Resources Development Act and the 1983 Social Security Amendments. The results of the study show that there were no changes in abnormal returns for the 1974 legislation. There was, however, a statistically significant reduction of 1.5% in the affected firms' stock market value following the 1983 Social Security Amendments. It should be noted, however, that the effects of the 1983 legislation was only minimal.

The second study addresses the effects of the U.S. Environmental Protection Agency's (EPA) efforts to reduce the risk of radon exposure by the population through education, testing, and mitigation activities. The study

Proven Solutions for Improving Health and Lowering Health Care Costs, pages 11–30.
Copyright © 2003 by Information Age Publishing, Inc.
All rights of reproduction in any form reserved.
ISBN: 1-59311-000-6 (paper), 1-59311-001-4 (cloth)

was done by using a Projection Model which assesses how sensitive death rates are to a change in radon policy via testing or mitigation. The simulation model looks at four risk groups and exposure pathways. It looks for distribution of radon risk across the population. The results show that one third of the mortality associated with radon exposure is attributed to smokers and is therefore unavoidable. The remaining two thirds of mortalities is generated by the entire population; individuals are at minimal risk. Hence extensive radon reduction efforts are not warranted. Specific high exposure areas need the focus for radon mitigation.

The third study addresses the effect of Medicaid on the use of health care services. The research showed that the Medicaid Program has seen increased usage of health care services from the poorer populations. Since there are still barriers to Medicaid access to some of the poorer segments of the population, it is imperative that Medicaid programs need to keep their focus on removing barriers to access for at-risk populations.

The fourth study looks at the trends in health care research and development (R&D) activities and technology innovation. The study focused on national investment in health-related research, on approvals of new drugs by the U.S. Food and Drug Administration (FDA), and on the number of new products in the pipeline. The study showed that health R&D spending as a share of total R&D spending has significantly increased from 1986 to 1995. Time for FDA approvals of drugs has significantly improved when comparing the early 1990s with the late 1990s. And new products in the pipeline also show robust growth. The change that has also taken place is the source of funding for all the above research; private funding has taken up the slack generated by public funding, raising the issue of potentially a weakened basic health research environment.

The fifth study explores an overhaul of Medicare, in light of the uncertainties of future trends in the health care sector and the economic security of elderly and disabled beneficiaries. The analysis concludes that major changes in Medicare are not warranted at present (1999). It is interesting that two years later (2001) the pharmaceutical coverage for the elderly provided by Medicare was inadequate and needed to be expanded at significantly added cost to the Medicare system.

The sixth study addresses barriers to the implementation of clinical guidelines. The focus of the study was the clinical practice triage guidelines for unstable angina. The guidelines were proposed by the Agency for Healthcare Policy and Research (AHCPR). The guidelines were developed on the basis of over 10,000 emergency room cases where symptoms of acute cardiac ischemia were apparent. The study explores a number of weaknesses in the AHCPR triage guidelines. The author suggests that more participation by providers and clinicians is necessary for the development of a set of optimal clinical practice guidelines.

The seventh study addresses the stability of disability of enrollees in the program of all-inclusive care for the elderly (PACE). The PACE program is a national demonstration program of the Health Care Financing Administration (HCFA). The stability of disability found among PACE members suggests that the current payment method is appropriate. Studies of the general elderly population have shown significant improvements in functional status over time. However, PACE members tend to be older and more frail and thus in more need of care.

The eighth and final study covers the policy regarding medical records and privacy. The study examines the effect of study-specific consent requirements on observational research in a health environment. The study's focus was a Minnesota-based health plan where plan members were asked for their consent to participate in a specific study of the membership. The study revealed that requiring patient informed consent to gain access to medical records for a specific study is associated with a low participation rate. Low participation rates is problematic in epidemiological research because it compromises the ability to generalize from the results. So health policy requiring patient consent for research participation tends to inhibit the quality of the information that can be obtained from the research.

In this chapter we have reviewed a number of effects and implications of federal and state health policy on availability of services, effectiveness of care, protection of individuals, and quality of results obtained from research.

2.1 CAN INVESTORS PREDICT THE EFFECTS OF HEALTH POLICY?

Health care cost containment has been an area of concern to Congress for the past several decades. Pressure by employers who pay the bulk of health care costs of their employees through company-paid (wholly or partially) health insurance plans has been the primary impetus for these efforts at health care cost containment by Congress.

Researcher Carol K. Jacobson of Arizona State University and University of Western Australia (1994) studied the effects of two pieces of health care cost containment legislation on the stock market performance of health system firms which might be adversely affected by these two pieces of legislation. She hypothesized that if the stock market performance of the firms did not change, then the market anticipated the failure of the legislation.

The two pieces of legislation consisted of the National Health Planning and Resources Development Act of 1974 and the Social Security Amendments of 1983. The first act imposed mandatory state health planning programs to control duplication of health services in geographic areas. The second act intended to stimulate market competition as the driving force for cost control through the prospective payment system for hospital care.

Event study was used to evaluate the stock market performances for the 20 firms used in the study. In event study the firm's stock performance on the day following the legislation announcement is compared with the historical performance of the respective stock. Any differences are referred to as abnormal returns. The included firms consisted of direct providers of health services, distributors of professional hospital equipment, distributors of standard hospital supplies, and medical equipment manufacturers.

The results of the study indicated that there was no change in abnormal returns for the first event, the National Health Planning and Resources Development (NHPRD) Act. For the second event, the Social Security (SS) Amendments, a statistically significant reduction of 1.5 percent in the firms' returns was revealed. In other words the stock market investors did not feel threatened by the NHPRD Act, but showed concern for the SS Amendments, which introduced competition in the health care delivery system through a prospective payment system for hospital care.

To measure the impact of income growth for the preceding two years, financial leverage and firm size on abnormal returns at the event times, a crossectional regression was performed. The results of the regression indicated that the NHPRD Act showed no statistically significant results. However, for the SS Amendments, the results were significant with income growth having a negative effect and firm size having a positive effect on abnormal returns. Financial leverage had no effect.

The study results indicate that the intentions of Congress to pass cost containment legislation through the two legislative pieces (events) were essentially thwarted. The investors in the firms realized it at the event time and concluded that both legislative pieces were ineffective. The NHPRD Act was essentially ignored by investors. The SS Amendment resulted in an overall decline of 1.5 percent in abnormal returns indicating some concern on the part of the investors but no major concern.

The author attributes the results of the study to the impact of lobbying activities by affected parties to weaken both pieces of legislation so as to render them either much weaker than intended or ineffective to achieve the intended results. Such organizations as the American Hospital Association, the American Medical Association, and the American Association of Retired Persons may well have achieved at least part of their goals. In retrospect we have observed the relatively minor impact of the NHPRD Act, but the same cannot be said for the SS Amendments.

2.2   ASSESSING A FEDERAL ENVIRONMENT POLICY: THE EFFECT OF RADON

The United States Environmental Protection Agency targets radon exposure as a leading cause of lung cancer in the United States. EPA's strategy for reducing risk of radon exposure to the public is through education, testing, and mitigation activities. Mitigation activities consist of reducing or eliminating exposure to radon gas. In order to determine the strategy's effectiveness, EPA needs to know whether significant changes in mortality and even public response will be high enough to justify a public health policy.

Through his research, Michael Peterson (1996) attempts to evaluate the effectiveness of potential EPA radon policies by examining the likely impact they would have on public health when combined with public response. Past studies of radon exposure had mostly focused on the epidemiological aspects and on historical policy. Other researchers have presented an analysis of radon risk and impact on current mortality rates. However, Peterson takes research and data one step further and attempts to make projections on the effectiveness of using alternative radon policies over time.

Two complex mathematical models, the Projection Model and the Simulation Model, were created and a large amount of data were computed to address the two main issues. The Projection Model consists of three components, and assesses how sensitive radon death rates are to a change in radon policy via testing or mitigation. The first component, the Compartmental submodel, evaluates changes in housing stock over time. The second component, an Epidemiological submodel, takes into account changes in lung cancer mortality rates. The Actuarial submodel component translates changes into total mortalities. The Simulation Model looks at four risk groups and a total of 10,000 possible exposure pathways. This model allows for distribution of radon risk across the population.

The Projection Model research confirms past research results that show that current and former smokers account for the largest share of radon risk. The models show that a tripling of the public's mitigation response rate only reduces the mortality rate by less than ten percent. Research also shows that the number of radon-attributable lung cancer deaths remains relatively stable regardless of which policy is in effect. The reasoning behind this is that there is a wide distribution of exposures. Other observations show that because of the distribution effect, only large changes in public response will result in a significant reduction in mortalities. Evidence shows that there is a substantial decrease in mortalities if mitigation exceeds 23% for all homes designated Category I. Lastly, the Projection Model results show three significant theoretical outcomes. It appears that approximately 1/3 of radon lung cancers is unavoidable. The results show that current technology and behavior do not reach projections established by Congress. Reductions in smoking habits prove to have more impact on radon-related mortalities than policy itself.

The Simulation Model takes a different approach, and that is to distribute the radon risk across the entire population. The research results expose the fact that often times radon exposure is not limited to a single location. This oversight can be somewhat justified in that many moves are within a region that contains similar levels of radon exposure. In addition, this model takes into account that homes are usually occupied by more than one individual, and therefore the risk is distributed further. The costs and benefits of mitigation are also calculated by this model.

The results show that one-third of the mortality associated with radon exposure is attributed to smokers, and is therefore unavoidable. Public policy is targeted at the remaining two-thirds, which is a large population with small risk. It is determined that the high level of public response required for a substantial reduction in mortalities is unlikely to be achieved. The results do not suggest that all radon-reduction policies be eliminated, but argue that good management of low-cost strategies be pursued by the EPA. Such steps have already been taken with the "go-slow" strategy. Passive mitigation techniques in high risk areas are more cost effective than expensive testing and mitigation activities in all areas. Even in instances of moderate to high level public response, expensive policies and mitigation show a relatively small reduction in mortalities.

2.3   THE EFFECT OF MEDICAID ON HEALTH CARE SERVICES USE

Do Medicaid beneficiaries have the same access to health care as their similar uninsured and privately insured counterparts? In 1993 the Medicaid program paid for the health care of 13% of poor Americans at a cost of $125 billion. Because of this large expenditure, accurate estimates of effectiveness are necessary to determine the continued support and possible expansion of the Medicaid program. Past research has argued that Medicaid populations both continue to have barriers to access of proper health care and that they also use more health services than low-income private payers. Research is necessary to determine which of these diverse views is correct.

M. Susan Marquis and Stephen H. Long (1996), senior economists from RAND, a nonprofit institution that helps improve policy and decision-making through research and analysis, looked at the implications of Medicaid effectiveness. The researchers compared the health services use by similar populations of non-elderly adults and children covered by the AFDC (Aid to Families with Dependent Children) Medicaid program, the uninsured, and those covered by private insurance over the course of a year. The research was performed to gain accurate estimates of health care services use by Medicaid beneficiaries relative to what their use would be if they were uninsured or privately insured.

The researchers collected data from the 1987 National Medical Expenditure Survey (NMES) and the 1984-1988 Surveys of Income and Program Participation (SIPP). These surveys are two of the three major national sur-

veys focused on health services use that collect information from a representative population about each person's health, health care use,
insurance status, and economic and demographic characteristics. From
these surveys the researchers were able to restrict the samples to persons
under the age of 65, who received AFDC cash assistance. The low-income
elderly and patients with special health needs were part of these restrictions. These two groups have higher relative health services use compared
to other population groups because of their greater health care needs.

The research contrasts AFDC cash assistance Medicaid beneficiaries
continuously enrolled over a one-year period with similar uninsured or private insured individuals. Based on a prediction model, the annual utilization of ambulatory and inpatient hospital care for AFDC beneficiaries were
predicted so it could be compared with the annual use if they were uninsured or covered by private insurance. A two part model for each type of
care is used to predict health services use. The first part of each model
determines the probability of receiving that type of care, and the second
part of the model determines the total quantity of care for the users of the
service. (The number of ambulatory services, and the number of inpatient
hospital days.) Separate utilization models for adults (18-64 years of age)
and for children were used for age, sex, race and ethnicity, income as a
percentage of poverty, urban versus rural area, and self-reported health status. Insurance status, educational and marital status for adults, pregnancy,
and time trends were also captured indicators.

The model from each dataset was used to estimate health care use for
the AFDC beneficiaries and to predict, or simulate, each person's use if
they were uninsured or covered by private insurance. This model allows for
the measurement of the marginal effect of insurance, and the utilization
models are used to predict outcomes for the standard population. From
these models, the researchers were able to draw conclusions about health
care services usage by Medicaid beneficiaries.

The research concluded that the Medicaid program saw increased
usage of health care services among the poorer populations. The use
among the AFDC Medicaid beneficiaries proved to be similar to privately
insured persons. AFDC beneficiaries also had better ambulatory care
access (an increase of about 40%) than if they had remained uninsured.
However, there was a lower percentage of health care usage within the population than was expected. This conclusion suggests that there are still barriers of access to Medicaid beneficiaries for their needed health care.
Therefore, future expansion of the Medicaid program must include adequate access for at-risk populations, while keeping costs down.

Accurate estimates of use by Medicaid beneficiaries are essential in
deciding the effectiveness of the Medicaid program for improving health
care access for the poor. Some States are currently looking to expand the
program to groups of low-income individuals who were not previously eligible to participate, as there is concern that these individuals may experi-

ence difficulty in finding access to needed health care. These estimates are important to the State policymakers on projecting the costs and benefits of future expansions in the Medicaid program. Because of the high cost of the program, federal policymakers are also considering different options on controlling costs by limiting federal contributions to Medicaid by block grants to States and limits on federal payments per enrollee. Therefore, it is necessary for the States to show that the Medicaid program is successful and worth the investment for serving the poorer populations.

2.4   TECHNOLOGY INNOVATION IN HEALTH CARE RESEARCH AND DEVELOPMENT

Given the cost-conscious managed care environment, many analysts have expressed concern regarding the fate of health-related research and development (R&D). Their fear has been that the drive for efficiency might hinder the managed care plan's desire to pay for expensive drugs and technologies. Health R&D has steadily increased over the years, and the nation's overall commitment to R&D and innovation remains strong. The question raised then is who will pay for it?

Peter J. Neuman and Eileen Sandberg (1998), both of the Harvard School of Public Health, analyzed trends in three areas:

1. national investment in health-related research;
2. approvals of new drugs by the U.S. Food and Drug Administration FDA, and
3. new products in the pipeline.

This research was an update of an earlier study on funding for biomedical research and the pace of innovation in the pharmaceutical, medical device, and biotechnology industries.

Data concerning estimated national health expenditures for health care, total R&D, and health R&D was obtained from the National Institutes of Health (NIH). The NIH also provided information regarding support for R&D by source for the period 1986-1995, mean FDA approval times and number of new drug review applications submitted and the number of approved premarket approval applications. The Pharmaceutical Research and Manufacturers Association of America supplied the information regarding the number of AIDS drugs, total in development, and approved for the period 1987-1997.

National Investment in Health-Related Research

From 1986 to 1995 investment has increased, both in absolute terms and as a percent of total health care spending. In fact, health R&D spending as a share of total health R&D spending has significantly increased. The share of total health R&D within the industry has increased, as has industry R&D spending as a percentage of U.S. pharmaceutical sales.

FDA approval of new drugs

FDA approval time for new drugs and devices has decreased, due to several pieces of legislation, thus promoting a favorable climate for R&D. Although the number of new drugs approved in 1997 was down from 1996, the 1997 figure was still higher than the average for 1992-1995. Also, there was a significant increase in the total number of applications considered by the FDA. "Priority drugs" are so named due to their potential for significantly benefiting the recipient over other available therapies for serious illnesses. These are approved much more rapidly than non-priority drugs, and have been used in combating infection with HIV, AIDS, diabetes, atherosclerosis and osteoporosis. Also, the number of premarket approvals for medical devices has increased over the average level of 1992-1995.

Products in the pipeline

The number and types of diseases with drugs in clinical trials reflects the pace of development for new pharmaceutical sales. The most active clinical categories for new drugs in 1997 were cancer, AIDS, and heart disease and stroke. Another important trend in product development is biotechnology. Genomics research falls within this category. More than 30,000 human genes are now mapped and genes associated with various diseases are being sequenced. New companies are harnessing this expanding technology for developing a whole new level of drug development and medical care by aiding in the prediction, diagnosis, and treatment of inherited diseases.

Issues and Implications

While both the private and public sectors support a robust pace of R&D, several issues are evident. The data indicates a shift from public to private funding of R&D, which raises the question about whether enough basic research is being funded. Another area of concern is the ability of academic medical centers to subsidize clinical research. Also, attempts at reining in health costs through managed care may be overwhelmed by technology and drug costs. Another important question concerns who should pay for experimental treatments, the NIH, Medicare, or private insurers. Outcomes research needs to be expanded. Pharmacoeconomic analyses are now routinely done by drug companies and managed care plans now require economic evidence for new formulary submissions.

U.S. health care can be seen as a struggle between the nation's commitment to controlling costs versus its commitment to innovation. It seems that the biggest challenge remains determining who has access to the innovations and who pays for them.

2.5   MEDICARE OVERHAUL

The alarming increase in Medicare expenditures is creating calls for major reform of the federal Medicare program. On one side of the discussion are major deficits in funding for the program bringing into question future solvency of the Medicare trust fund. On the other side of the discussion are the needs of the baby boom generation as they approach retirement. Recent Medicare changes have assured trust fund solvency until 2007. A recent analysis of the situation suggests that future major changes in Medicare at this time are unwarranted.

Karen Davis (1999), President of the Commonwealth Fund in New York City, analyzed recent studies of Medicare beneficiaries and aging baby boomers in light of the enactment of the Balanced Budget Act. The analysis is based on a presentation at the Medicare Policy Roundtable sponsored by the Association of Health Services Research at their annual meeting on June 21, 1998. The analysis was also presented to the National Bipartisan Commission on the Future of Medicare at a hearing on "Medicare and Baby Boomers" on April 28, 1998, by invitation.

Her presentations concerned themselves with the uncertainty of future trends in the health care sector and the economic security of elderly and disabled beneficiaries. Of particular concern was the impact of baby boomers soon to be entering the Medicare program.

Future trends in the health care expenditures are determined by several factors. The first factor is the impact of future medical progress resulting from research in the biotechnology and pharmaceutical industries. The second factor concerns itself with changes in the health habits of older people. A third factor is the impact of the shift from an emphasis on institutional care to an emphasis on outpatient care. Another factor is the certainty of current economic projections. The analysis reviewed each of these factors.

Similar to future trends, the economic security of elderly and disabled beneficiaries is also determined by several factors. The first factor is the proportion of health care costs paid by Medicare beneficiaries. A second factor is the impact of health coverage provided by the retiree's former employer. The third factor concerns risks shouldered by low-income beneficiaries. A fourth factor concerns the disproportionate share of expenditures incurred by the sickest beneficiaries. Another major factor to be considered is the transition of Medicare from fee-for-service to managed care plans. The analysis reviewed these factors as well.

The analysis concludes that major changes in the Medicare program are unwarranted at this time. Since the Balanced Budget Act (BBA) has extended solvency of the Medicare trust fund, the analysis suggests that we take some time to implement and assess the impact of BBA on projected Medicare expenditures. The result of this assessment should then be utilized to assure trust fund solvency and security for elderly and disabled beneficiaries.

This analysis bases this conclusion on the fact that the results of future trends are unknowable. Additionally, the economic security of the elderly and disabled beneficiaries is very much in question.

Future trends are not factored into the solvency projections of the Medicare program. Research indicates that the prospect of significant advances in the ability to intervene in some of today's major causes of death and disability (i.e. cancer, heart disease, and Alzheimer's) is encouraging. Baby boomers will be better educated, less likely to smoke, and more active physically and mentally. Reliance on specialty care is decreasing and excess health care system capacity is beginning to shrink. Evaluating whether productivity is on the rise, the retirement age will stop declining, or what the immigration trends will be will impact payroll tax revenues. The answers to these uncertainties should be better known and factored into solvency projections.

The analysis suggests that changes in the Medicare program should be incremental (e.g., every five years) and we should gauge their effect before making more changes. The analysis suggests that the following three effects be assessed periodically.

- The financial burden on beneficiaries from premiums and out of pocket expenses and the impact on access to care.
- The ability of the healthcare sector to absorb Medicare savings without deterioration in the quality of care.
- The extent to which Medicare payment rates for both fee-for-service providers and managed care plans are competitive with the private sector.

The economic security of elderly and disabled beneficiaries is very much in question. The growth of Medicare outlays per beneficiary is staggering. The health care costs that beneficiaries pay themselves are high and growing just as rapidly. Currently, beneficiaries pay 37% of their own health care cost not including Medicare Part B premiums. Prescription drugs and long-term care are the most rapidly increasing costs for beneficiaries.

One of the popular misconceptions is that all older people have retiree health coverage to supplement Medicare. In 1988, 44 percent of retirees had coverage from a previous employer. In 1994, only 30 percent have this coverage. This trend is likely to continue.

Most Medicare beneficiaries have modest or low incomes. Three-quarters have incomes below $25,000. Forty percent have incomes below 200 percent of the poverty level or about $15,400 in 1997. Medicaid covers some of the gap but not all. Various subsidy programs cover some but not all. Poor and chronically ill beneficiaries are particularly vulnerable. The health of these beneficiaries is especially at risk.

Averages used to project Medicare outlays mask a wide variation in health outlays for Medicare beneficiaries. The sickest 10 percent of beneficiaries account for 75 percent of Medicare outlays. This is especially important for Medicare payments per beneficiary to private plans. It may be necessary to consider a blended approach that combines prospective payments with capitation in order to reduce incentives to deny needed care to the sickest.

Enrollment in Medicare managed care plans is likely to accelerate with passage of BBA. Expanded managed care enrollment is likely to increase Medicare costs. The actual cost of serving Medicare beneficiaries in managed care plans is 5.7 percent higher than Medicare would have paid under fee-for-service. This is due to administrative costs in managed care of 10 to 12 percent versus 2 percent for Medicare. BBA reduces the rate of increase in payments to managed care plans. The impact of this provision should be evaluated.

Considering the impact of all these influences on the economic security of elderly and disabled beneficiaries is necessary. Additionally, Medicare payment rates must be comparable to payment rates in the private sector. The reason is to ensure continued access to necessary care. Differences in age of those covered and variations in benefit packages must be factored into this comparison.

The analysis has many implications in the business community. It is important to address the adequacy of the benefit package and protection for the most vulnerable beneficiaries—those who are low income and seriously ill. Medicare will need to adapt as the health system changes. The Medigap supplemental insurance market will come under increasing pressure as healthier beneficiaries enroll in managed care. Finding a way to capture the advantages of choice and competition without losing the purpose of Medicare will be a major future challenge.

2.6   BARRIERS TO CLINICAL GUIDELINES IMPLEMENTATION

One of the concerns of the medical care community is quality of care provided to patients. When assessing quality it has been discovered that great variation in practice patterns exists from region to region and from physician to physician. The result has been the proliferation of guidelines on patient care. The purpose of clinical guidelines is to standardize care provided and assure the best possible outcome for the patient. To a large extent these guidelines have fallen short of their intended purpose. What are the barriers preventing successful implementation of clinical guidelines?

David A. Katz, M.D., M.Sc. (1999) with the support of the Robert Wood Johnson Generalist Physician Faculty Scholars Program and institutional funds, undertook a study to identify the barriers to successful guideline implementation. Dr. Katz is on the staff of the Department of Medicine at the University of Wisconsin Madison.

For the study, Dr. Katz emphasized the recommendations for triage in the Agency for Health Care Policy and Research (AHCPR) Unstable Angina Clinical Practice Guideline. The guideline resulted from a prospective clinical study of 10,785 patients presenting to the emergency department with symptoms suggestive of acute cardiac ischemia.

The study is an analysis of the AHCPR guideline with regard to recognized barriers to guideline implementation. This was accomplished through presentation of hypothetical scenarios to emergency department physicians to determine reliability in applying the guideline to assess risk and make triage decisions.

The study analyzed the AHCPR Unstable Angina Clinical Guideline in light of the seven recognized barriers to achieving the objectives of guidelines. These seven recognized barriers are:

1. Excessive complexity and difficulty in testing the guideline in practice
2. Limited applicability
3. Failure to capture subtle clinical nuances that make a guideline inappropriate
4. Poor quality scientific evidence
5. Unexpected effects on other aspects of medical care
6. Organizational inefficiencies that impede guideline effectiveness
7. Unpredictable effects of local adaptation

The guideline calls for initial triage of patients with unstable angina based on risk factors for poor short-term outcome. High-risk patients are admitted to an intensive care bed. Intermediate risk patients are admitted to a telemetry or intensive care bed. Low risk patients are referred to outpatient management with close follow-up. The guideline's intention is to prevent unnecessary hospital admission of low risk patients to an intensive care or telemetry bed in a hospital. The results of Dr. Katz's study of this guideline follow.

Complexity and Reliability

The guideline is highly complex and difficult to pretest because integrating relevant criteria required for risk stratification of these patients is a challenging task. Emergency department physicians given clinical situations characteristic of intermediate and low risk groups were unable to properly use the guideline. A strategy to improve guideline reliability may be to present the guideline in an alternative format, such as a clinical algorithm or critical pathway.

Applicability

The guideline clearly defines the target population and provides useful evidence-based recommendations regarding management of unstable angina patients. However, evaluation of the triage portion revealed that only 6 percent of patients were at low risk and eligible for outpatient management. This suggests that reductions in hospitalization of patients would be modest. However, potential savings on a national level would be substantial.

Failure to Capture Subtle Clinical Nuances

The guideline captures many subtleties in clinical presentation for predicting predict short-term outcome. However, it fails to account explicitly for influences of other medical, psychiatric, or social problems that may indicate deviation from its triage recommendations. Guidelines should demonstrate clinical flexibility by identifying specific or generally expected exceptions to their recommendations.

Unexpected Effects on Other Aspects of Medical Care

Based on evaluation of actual versus recommended disposition, it was determined that 60 percent of high-risk patients were triaged to telemetry rather than intensive care. Strict adherence would require intensive care admission even though there was no compelling reason to do so. Thus, while the guideline is intended to reduce unnecessary hospitalization, the effect may lead to significant increases in demand for limited intensive care beds.

Poor Quality Scientific Evidence

Triage recommendations in the guideline were based largely on observational studies and expert opinion. Even with this limitation their evaluation indicated that the guideline effectively stratified patients across multiple dimensions. However, the risk groups specified by the guideline did not improve identification of patients with suspected heart attacks when compared to physician judgement. Additionally, the guideline's impact on patient outcomes has yet to be demonstrated.

Organizational Inefficiencies that Impede Guideline Effectiveness

The guideline encourages hospitals to discharge low-risk emergency department patients and provides for outpatient follow-up within 48-72 hours of initial presentation. In the study hospitals' policies were in place that recommended admission for patients who were admitted to the emergency department with stable angina. Under the guideline these low-risk patients would be discharged home from the emergency department. Successful implementation of the guideline requires admission to an intensive care bed for high-risk patients. In the study hospitals there was no intensive care bed available for 25 percent of these patients. Therefore, significant organizational barriers exist in guideline implementation.

Unpredictable Effects of Local Adaptation

The effect of modifying a guideline to conform to local beliefs and systems of care are often unpredictable. Few studies have specifically addressed this topic. This study is no exception.

Recent experience indicates that developing sound, evidence-based guidelines is not enough to improve the quality of health care. Careful attention to both knowledge based and organizational factors in the implementation process will maximize the possibility of improving patient care. When attempting to provide high quality patient care in the appropriate setting under ever-increasing revenue constraints, providers and clinicians must collaborate in the development and implementation of clinical care guidelines.

2.7   STABILITY OF ELDERLY PATIENTS IN A HOME CARE PROGRAM

Managed long-term care programs often base their premium rates on the assumption that disability is a permanent condition for their enrollees and they therefore maintain constant premium rates for this population. Programs called "Program of All-inclusive Care for the Elderly" (PACE) are designed to provide preventive, primary, acute, and long term services to nursing home certifiable persons who choose to stay in the community. PACE is a national demonstration program of the Health Care Financing Administration (HCFA) and uses a health status-based modification to the Medicare health maintenance organization (HMO) rate, the adjusted average per capita cost (AAPCC). This creates a higher Medicare payment for its participants, all of whom are nursing home certifiable, and are therefore expected to have higher expenditures than other enrollees. Although the AAPCC is an adjustment to the HMO rate, the AAPCC is the same for all PACE enrollees, regardless of their functional status, and is not updated over time. Eleven PACE programs have been developed since 1990. While many studies have examined the progress of disability among general elderly populations, only two studies have evaluated changes in disability for the PACE population. Is disability among PACE enrollees permanent? Are HMOs being paid appropriately by Medicare and Medicaid for this population?

These questions were examined in a study by Dana Mukamel (1998) of the University of Rochester, Helena Temkin-Greener of ViaHealth and the Community Coalition for Long-Term Care, and Marlene Clark of On Lok, Inc., San Francisco. The authors investigated the stability of disability for PACE enrollees over time and the financial implications of this. Also, the authors looked for characteristics on admission to the program which were associated with improvement or deterioration.

PACE data on 2,291 individuals from eleven PACE sites located in eight States, all fully capitated since 1992, were used in this retrospective exploratory study. A time series analysis ending at 18 months after enrollment focused on change in functional status in relation to enrollment as well as on the effect of individual risk factors on the probability of change in that period. The five possible functional outcomes were: death, disenrollment, no change, improvement, or deterioration. Risk factors associated with change in functional status were identified by modeling the probability of the five possible outcomes as a function of all risk factors present on admission.

Stability of Disability

After 18 months over half of the enrollees remained at the same level of disability. About a fourth improved or deteriorated, with the amount of those improving being slightly higher than those who deteriorated and another 13 percent had died. The probability of improving was greatest in the first three months, after which the probability of change was very low.

Effect of Individual Risk Factors on Changes in Disability Level

The risk factors found to be significant predicators of change in disability status included the following: A limitation in bathing oneself was a strong predictor of improvement, probably because it was an activity most likely to respond to PACE interventions. Urinary incontinence and dementia both lowered the probability of improvement. Contrary to current thought on the subject, enrollees who live alone had better outcomes than those living with others. In fact, by 18 months they were almost twice as likely to improve as those living with others.

Business Implications

The stability of disability found in this study suggests that the current payment method is appropriate. Little, if anything, is to be gained financially from periodic readjustments for PACE enrollees. While studies of the general elderly population have shown significant improvement in functional status over time, PACE enrollees tend to be older and more frail. Factors associated with improvement or deterioration need to be further explored, in order to identify opportunities for improving care and outcomes.

2.8   LEGISLATIVE EFFECTS ON MEDICAL RECORDS PRIVACY

The public's concern regarding privacy in this computer and technology era is bringing about legislative proposals to strengthen existing confidentiality protections for patient medical records and information. The question that rises is how to balance societal values which respect individual privacy and are vital to patient trust in the health care process *and* simultaneously allow access to information that is essential for scientific research to improve health and health care for the society as a whole? There is little information available to date which addresses this concern for policy considerations.

Proposed individual privacy protections affecting research are intended to ensure that access to medical records bears in mind patient autonomy, heeds patient confidentiality, and serves a socially valued purpose. The idea of informed consent is a long-standing ethical protection for human-subject research involving an intervention or interaction that risks harm to an individual. However, the use of existing medical records and information for observational research poses no risk of physical harm or minimal risk to privacy. Current Federal Policy for the Protection of Human Subjects exempts retrospective medical record research when the patient is not identified. However, when research is subject to review by an institutional board, an informed consent may be required.

Some argue that use of any medical records without consent constitutes a breach of trust. In support of this view a poll found that 64% of these respondents objected to the use of their medical records for research without their consent. Others argue that obtaining consent to use medical records is not always feasible and a delay may harm the public by impeding important health research. In other words, society must decide whether benefits of health research outweigh the intrusion of privacy if there is adequate confidentiality protection.

The researchers, McCarthy, Shatin, and Drinkard of the Center for Health Care Policy and Evaluation in Minneapolis, Minnesota, Kleinman of Allina Health System, and Gardner of Pharmaceutical Outcomes Research Policy at the University of Washington (1999), examine the effect of a study-specific consent requirement on observational research in the health plan environment.

The case study was a pharmaco-epidemiologic study to determine the risk of seizure associated with the use of a newly marketed oral analgesic medication as a postmarketing surveillance effort to determine the severity of adverse events associated with the approved drug. The results of such studies assist the FDA in determining whether additional warnings or restrictions are warranted to help avoid unwanted treatment consequences and have potentially significant public health implications for ensuring the use of prescription drugs safely.

The method to accomplish the objective of the study is as follows. A large Minnesota based IPA's administrative claims were used which included pharmacy, medical, and enrollment files, and medical records from physician offices and hospitals. A cohort of 9,377 users and 37,367 non-users of the oral analgesic were identified and seizure outcomes were distinguished by claims from each group. The user group's medical records were utilized to collect information regarding potential confounding risk factors such as head injury or stroke, which might account for the seizure occurrence.

The Minnesota health plan was subject to the State's informed consent requirement. A letter was sent out to the members of the identified cohort requesting participation. The members were asked to sign and return the form indicating whether or not they wished to authorize access to their medical records for the study. A second letter was sent six weeks later making the same request to those whom did not respond to the first letter. Then follow-up phone calls were made to those who did not respond to either letter encouraging them to return the consent form.

Thirty-one percent, after the first request letter was sent, responded with a signed consent form. Fourteen percent authorized access to medical records, and 17 percent declined authorization to access. After the second request letter, an additional 2 percent authorized access while an additional 7 percent denied access. The follow-up phone calls resulted in an additional 3 percent authorizing access and another 10 percent denying access. The cumulative grand total was 19 percent authorization and 34 percent declining authorization with no responses by 47 percent. In another State where study-specific consent is not required, health care providers granted access to patient medical records for 93 percent of the members based on a general enrollment authorization.

This study reveals that requiring patient informed consent to gain access to medical records for a specific study is associated with a low participation rate in the study. Low participation is problematic in epidemiological research because it compromises the ability to generalize from the results. In other words those who decline access or fail to respond altogether may be different in a clinically significant way from those who did authorize use of their records in such a way that may not be representative of the entire study population. Those who have experienced a seizure may be hesitant to participate if they fear consequences such as loss of driving privileges or insurance discrimination. In addition to this, the time and effort required to gain consent in this study did not increase the participation rate appreciably.

There is obvious tension between protecting the public health and protecting patient privacy. This study implies that legislation requiring informed consent for medical record access for specific studies may have unintended consequences on the ability of researchers to conduct observational research. The societal implication is derived from the fact that health care delivery environments offer vital advantages for conducting population-based research while allowing for timely evaluation of health effects and the associated service utilization to the general health of the community.

REFERENCES

Davis, K. (1999). Shaping the future of Medicare. *Health Services Research, 34*(1, Part 2, Supplement), 295-306.

Jacobson, C.K. (1994). Investor response to health care cost containment legislation: Is American health policy designed to fail? *Academy of Management Journal, 37*(2), 440-452.

Katz, D. A. (1999). Barriers between guidelines and improved patient care: An analysis of AHCPR's unstable angina clinical practice guideline. *Health Services Research, 34*(1, Part 2 Supplement), 377-389.

Marquis, M. S., & Long, S. H. (1996). Reconsidering the effect of medicaid on health care services use. *Health Services Research, 30*(6), 791-809.

McCarthy, D. B., Shatin, D., Drinkard, C. R., Kleinman, J. H., & Gardner, J. S. (1999). Medical records and privacy: Empirical effects of legislation. *Health Services Research, 34*(1), 417-423.

Mukamel, D. B., Temkin-Greener, H., & Clark, M. (1998) Stability of disability among PACE enrollees: Financial and programmatic implications. *Health Care Financing Review, 19*(3), 83-100.

Neuman P. J., & Sandberg, E. A. (1998). Trends in health care R&D and technology innovation. *Health Affairs*, (November-December), 111-119.

Peterson, M. D. (1996). Two models for assessing a federal environmental health policy: The case of radon in U.S. homes. *Management Science, 42*(10), 1476-1492.

CHAPTER 3

HEALTH ECONOMICS

In this chapter we cover the topic of economics and health care. Such topics as monopsony power, economic impact, internal labor market, competition versus legislation, cost of obesity, etc. are covered in this chapter.

The first study discusses monopsony power and relative wages in the labor market for registered nurses. Monopsony power is explored in this context because despite wide shortages, there have been no concomitant increases in wages for registered nurses. The researchers tested their theory by using a collusion model. A collusion model tests for the degree of collusion among employers to limit high wages. Collusion was not found and thus the monopsony theory had to be rejected. Yet, there remains a shortage of nurses. The authors hypothesize that it may be caused by the increase in the elderly population and in the need for more registered nurses to deal with the high technology employed in acute medical care.

The second study addresses the economic impact of Piperacillin/Tazobactam in the treatment of suspected polymicrobial infections. Piperacillin/Tazobactam (PZ) is an expensive antibiotic that has the ability to eliminate bacteria that cannot be eliminated with lower-cost antibiotics. The study aims to prove that the PZ antibiotic is more beneficial despite its higher cost. The research results indicated that the clinical use of the PZ antibiotic in the treatment of lower respiratory and intra-abdominal infections is cost-effective.

Proven Solutions for Improving Health and Lowering Health Care Costs, pages 31–46.
Copyright © 2003 by Information Age Publishing, Inc.
All rights of reproduction in any form reserved.
ISBN: 1-59311-000-6 (paper), 1-59311-001-4 (cloth)

The third study is a labor market study. Its title is cost, commitments, and rewards—factors influencing the design and implementation of internal labor markets: The study is a three-part case study covering a manufacturing firm, a consulting firm, and a hospital. The research results among the three organizations revealed that internal labor markets are related to both external markets and organizational hierarchies. External markets dictate what skills are available and what the costs of acquiring (wages) these skills are. There is also the cost of searching, evaluating, hiring, and training new hires. Within the firms there are hierarchies. These hierarchies involve the training and other overhead costs of retraining current employees. The two higher skilled firms, the consulting firm (trained and experienced consultants) and the hospital (trained registered nurses) both found that it is cheaper to retrain staff than to recruit new staff.

The fourth study describes mental health care and provider choice. The study examines the ways in which the costs of non-residential mental health care depends on the type of provider who initiates the treatment episode and the level of cost sharing with the patient. The objective of the study was to determine if both patient and provider influence the type and cost of the mental health therapy. Research results indicate that out-of-pocket costs significantly affect the patient's initial choice of provider type, but after provider type is selected the effectiveness of the therapy is indifferent to provider type.

The fifth study addresses the controversial question if competition or government regulation will constrain the spiraling health care expenditures. The study analyzed statistical data related to hospital discharge costs in the 15 States with the highest HMO penetration. To compare States with different economic and demographic conditions the hospital discharge rates were adjusted for case mix severity and the Medicare wage index. Adjustments were also made for medical education type expenses and hospitalization per capita rates. The results indicate that higher HMO market penetration does not per se result in lower hospitalization costs. Either relative inefficiency of the State-managed hospital reimbursement rates or high hospital discharge rates can contribute to high per capita hospitalization costs. Annual growth of reimbursement rates was much higher than the inflation rates in all of the States suggesting need for cost containment efforts.

The sixth study explores the cost of obesity in the USA. The study attempts to estimate the direct and indirect costs of obesity-associated disease in the USA in the year 1990. The economic costs include health care-related costs and the cost of work days lost and mortality costs based on lifetime earnings lost. The four main areas of health-related costs included gallbladder disease ($3.2 billion), cardiovascular disease ($29.4 billion), cancer ($0.7 billion) and musculoskeletal disease ($3.8 billion). Clearly the overwhelming cost item is cardiovascular disease. Indirect costs included work days lost ($4 billion) and mortality ($19 billion). Another contributor to the cost of obesity was diabetes, amounting to about $10 billion for a total cost of about $70 billion.

The seventh study reviews the cost and financing of care for persons with HIV disease. The estimate of the Center for Disease Control and Prevention (CDC) estimates the number of HIV disease cases in 1996 to amount to 650,000–900,000. The new drug therapies provide a longer and better quality of life for HIV disease patients, but the new treatments also add significant costs. And as HIV disease sufferers live longer they consume more health care resources, further increasing the expenditures for the HIV disease. One additional benefit of the new drug therapies is a lowering of hospitalization rates. The conclusion of the study was that HIV disease treatment will continue to rise in the future.

The eighth and final study looks at the future for primary care financing. The study focuses on the benefits of the primary care provider serving as the gatekeeper to limit or manage the patient's access to specialty care. The database used is the American Medical Association's (AMA) Socioeconomic Monitoring System (SMS) to evaluate managed care penetration and the changes in physician income. The results of the study show that for one percentage point increase in managed care penetration, primary care physicians gained $2263 in real income, subspecialty physicians gained $530 and radiologists, anesthesiologists and pathologists lost $1993. As a result the study found a significant increase in the incomes of primary care physicians in States with high managed-care growth. It will be interesting to see how the weakening of the gatekeeper system in the late 1990s has affected the income levels of the various physician groups.

This chapter has covered a number of interesting economic studies of health issues. The most notable are the high cost to society of obesity and HIV disease, the potential savings by using lower cost providers for mental health therapy, and several labor market issues.

3.1   IS THERE COLLUSION IN SETTING SALARY LEVELS FOR NURSES?

Researchers have paid considerable attention to the labor market for nurses. This attention results from the purported shortages that have appeared periodically in nursing labor markets. Monopsony could help explain shortages since hospitals will actively recruit nurses in an effort to hire additional nurses at monopsonistic and low wages as opposed to raising wages to attract nurses thus increasing labor costs. Recent research has found that there is no positive relationship between the monopsony model and relative nursing wages, hospital density, or market size.

Researchers Barry T. Hirsch, Florida State University, Tallahassee, Florida, and Edward J. Schumacher, East Carolina University, Greenville, North

Carolina (1995), examined the thesis that monopsony power is an important determinant of wages in nursing labor markets. A model was constructed using data from the 1985-1993 Current Population Surveys, a
measure of relative nurse / non-nurse wage rates for 252 labor markets.

One test of the theory was a collusion model. For example if hospitals or
other large employers acted in collusion or "cooperation" to limit wages
and employment to a level which maximizes joint profits or minimize joint
costs, then potentially a monopsonistic outcome may be achieved. However, if employers do not cooperate and try to attract labor from their competitors, and enough employers operate this way, a competitive outcome
will result.

Empirical testing of monopsony required the determination of whether
wages in a labor market are low relative to a counterfactual competitive
outcome along with a measure of market characteristics such as size and
number of employers. Nursing samples included all hospital and non-hos-
pital registered nurses, licensed practical nurses and nurses aids. Control
groups were constructed including all female workers meeting similar criteria, with a wide occupational background. This group was broken down
into three distinct groups based on education. By measuring nursing wages
relative to the control groups, measurable worker and market characteristics could be controlled.

A two step estimation procedure was used to test for monopsony effects
on wage. First, area-specific nursing wage differentials for the 252 areas
were estimated, where the differential represented the difference between
nursing and non-nursing wages in that labor market taking into account
measurable characteristics. Second, the nursing / non-nursing differentials were examined for variability with labor market characteristics across
but not within areas.

Little support is found for the monopsony model. Contrary to predictions, wages of nursing personnel are not related to hospital density, and
tend to decrease rather than increase with respect to labor market size.
Absence of statistically significant differences in wages between urban and
non-urban areas, and the relationship of relative wage and hospital density
suggest that monopsony power is limited. Even though the study discounts
the validity of a monopsony hypothesis, there is the unexplained chronic
shortage of registered nurses in the labor market. This may result from the
growing elderly population and the demand for an increase in nurses per
hospital bed to complement more sophisticated medical technologies.

This study has provided insight into the recent wage determination for
the nursing workforce across labor markets of various size along with econ-
omy-wide control groups. This may assist in the decision making process
for the establishment of wage, incentive, and quality expectations during
the hiring of nurses in a tight labor market. This also leads one to expect
that in an economically depressed area shortages of nurses are to be

expected, resulting from relative ease of relocating to other labor markets without compromising wage and working conditions.

3.2 ECONOMIC IMPACT OF USING A HIGHER-PRICED DRUG IN THE TREATMENT OF INFECTIONS?

In recent years, and for various reasons, the effectiveness of many broad-spectrum intravenous antibiotics has been lessened. This problem is of major concern, not only to the cost-conscious healthcare industry, but also to the overall health of the world population, which seems to be losing the bacterial infection wars.

One problem specifically diminishes the ability of the popular beta-lactam class of antibiotics to do their job. Some strains of bacteria, which have been exposed to these antibiotics for decades now, have developed the ability to defend themselves by producing chemicals that render the drugs useless. The bacteria, sensing the presence of a beta-lactam antibiotic, emit beta-lactamases, which dismantle the molecular chain of the antibiotic. These resistant bacteria have been particularly lethal to already compromised patients hospitalized with lower respiratory and intra-abdominal infections.

To combat the prevalence of these beta-lactamase producing bugs, researchers Daniel M. Huse, Mason W. Russell, Shelley Drowns, David R. Snydman, and Stuart C. Hartz (1998) have evaluated a new class of drugs, called beta-lactamase inhibitors, to the standard beta-lactam antibiotics. In the attempt to bolster the use of one such antibiotic combination, piperacillin sodium/tazobactam sodium, and to justify its higher cost per dose, the researchers in this study hoped to show a positive economic impact from using this drug on certain infections in US hospitals.

This study is based on data from a multicenter, randomized, controlled clinical trial conducted at three hospitals in the US. Patients were hospitalized with either community-acquired lower respiratory tract infections, hospital-acquired lower respiratory tract infections, or intra-abdominal infections. Patients were either given Piperacillin/tazobactam at its proper dose, or given what is considered to be the accepted drug of choice for their given infection.

In the community-acquired lower respiratory tract infection evaluation, 114 patients were randomized to receive piperacillin/tazobactam (P/T), while 74 were given ticarcillin (T/C). Per-patient costs of treatment with P/T and T/C were \$295 and \$247, respectively. However, P/T patients required fewer doses, spent less time in special care units, and were discharged earlier. Therefore, total costs of hospitalization were \$2981 lower per patient in the P/T group.

In the hospital-acquired lower respiratory infection evaluation, 99 patients were randomized to receive P/T, while 91 were treated with ceftazidime (C). Per-patient costs of treatment with P/T and C were $802 and $639, respectively. Total costs of hospitalization for the P/T patients was $702 higher, not a desirable outcome for the researchers. However, fewer patients died in the P/T group.

In the intra-abdominal infection evaluation, 101 patients were randomized to P/T, while 45 were given Clindamycin plus Gentamicin (C/G). Per-patient costs were estimated to be $284 and $113, respectively. Almost all of this cost difference was offset by more frequent dosing and the need to add additional drugs to the treatment of the C/G group.

This data supports the clinical use of piperacillin sodium/tazobactam sodium in the treatment of lower respiratory and intra-abdominal infections and also supports its use when overall economic impact to hospitals is analyzed. Too often medical facilities make decisions on antibiotic usage largely on the per dose purchase price of the medications. This data shows the importance of analyzing the overall treatment costs associated with these medications. More often than not studies such as this one show that newer, more scientifically sound agents, such as P/T, while having a higher per dose cost, are more effective and, therefore, more economically beneficial than their older, less effective predecessors.

3.3   EFFECTIVENESS OF INTERNAL TRAINING VERSUS EXTERNAL HIRING

Internal Labor Markets (ILM) are the markets that exist within organizations and they comprise the way employees are hired, compensated, trained, and promoted. The research conducted in this article was geared towards understanding the way firms in the mid-1980s handled their internal labor markets. There was some apparent research conducted in this area, but there were problems that affected the firms' ILMs that were never addressed before. Therefore, these problems will become more extensive if firms do not recognize them. The two main problems that this research focuses on is the recession in the mid-1980's economy and a decrease in the number of skilled workers in the external labor market.

David Bills (1987) wanted to research internal labor markets for two reasons: there was no descriptive material showing the variations from ideal ILMs and there was limited knowledge on why firms want to internalize and maintain their internal labor markets instead of recruiting from the outside labor markets. In order to research ILMs, David Bills interviewed three organizations: Northside Manufacturing, Exurb Consulting, and City Hospital (nursing staff). He wanted to get the viewpoint on how a manufacturing, consulting, and a not-for-profit hospital made hiring and promotion decisions. These interviews were conducted with employees who were responsible for making the hiring and promotion decisions within their firms. The following will indicate how these firms differ on their hiring and promotion decisions.

Northside Manufacturing is a unionized firm that hires mainly skilled workers (tool and die makers, machinists, and production workers). The union is weak which allows management to have more control over the decision-making process. This company has very little formal promotion lines, career ladders, or career counseling. The only major structured advancement program at Northside is their apprenticeship program. Here workers can apply for the program and if selected through a testing program, they can advance through various apprentice levels. This program trains them to be journeypersons and gives them leverage for higher pay. The goal of the apprenticeship program is to retain employees. Northside has a very high turnover rate due to their low wages, even with the journeypersons. Bills noted that Northside needs to reconsider their wage rates since the supply of skilled labor in their area is very limited.

Exurb Consulting has a different way of handling their ILM. This is an engineering consulting firm for construction and public works projects. They have a career line for their engineers called the Eleven Disciplines. These disciplines reflect area of skill or expertise. This system allows for Exurb to reward employees without forcing them into management positions. This company did not want to rely on the external labor markets for engineering skills because they believe that engineering skills are highly specialized and the market for these skills are scarce in their area. Another program that Exurb is trying to implement is training their technicians to be engineers. The reason is that they feel that the consulting skills that the engineers need are not something that can be learned in school. These skills have to be learned on the job and through other engineers.

City Hospital also implemented an internal promotion program for their nurses. The program is divided into 4 clinicals (I, II, III, IV). Inexperienced nurses are hired into Clinical Nurse I and experienced nurses are hired into Clinical Nurse II. There are pay differences among these 2 groups. Clinical III and Clinical IV are never filled from the outside. These promotions are from the nurses within City Hospital. Clinical III and Clinical IV promotions allow the nurses to move into teaching, management, or research, whereby a formal mentoring program is established with each nurse promoted into these areas. The pay scale at this facility is very competitive with surrounding hospitals. The reason for this step program and having a competitive wage scale is to minimize the threat of unionization among their nurses.

The research results among the three organizations indicated that internal labor markets are the function of both external markets and hierarchies (within the organizations). External labor dictates what level of skills are available to firms and the wage rate that people with different skills are demanding. There is the cost of searching, recruiting, and training new hires. This cost is much higher for firms than hiring from within. On the other hand, there are the hierarchies that exist within these firms. These involve the training and overhead cost of retaining employees. The costs can be substantial to some firms, but as Exurb and City Hospital explained it is cheaper to retain than to recruit new hires.

After looking at economic considerations, the mid 1980s recession in the market affected the firms differently. Northside cut their training costs and laid off some of their workers. Northside figured that they could maintain skilled workers through their apprenticeship program because that program allows them to have a skilled workforce at a lower wage rate. Exurb maintained their ILM because they know there is a tight market for the engineers they are looking for. Exurb's system was viewed by their employees as a status system because engineers and technicians could advance to the next level. City Hospital knew that there was a surplus of nurses in their area and they also knew that they could raise the hiring standards in order to seek the most qualified nurses that best fit their organization. City Hospital did cut some training programs during the recession, but they were able to keep the highly skilled nurses with their competitive wages.

This research has many different implications for business in the area of employment. By studying various organizations and benchmarking them, you are able to understand which tactics they are using and why they have these programs. Many businesses can learn from this study on ways to retain workers without depending on the external labor force. This builds security and trust within organizations and it can, at times, suppress unionization. This study also shows that when there is more of a tight or a loose workforce, ILMs are important to firms. Organizations can raise their hiring standards when there are many workers fighting for skilled jobs, and firms can retain workers by using internal promotions and training when there are not many workers with those skills in the local area. It might take time and resources to build an ILM; however, the cost of recruiting and training new hires is far more expensive for most companies.

3.4   MENTAL HEALTH CARE AND PROVIDER CHOICE

This study examines the ways in which the costs of nonresidential mental health care depend on the type of provider who initiates the treatment episode and the level of cost sharing imposed on the patient. The magnitude and growth of costs has led to much debate about the optimal benefit design for mental health care insurance coverage, and the optimal organization's structure for the delivery of mental care.

The purpose of this article was to determine the extent to which patients and providers influence the patterns of mental health care use and the costs of treatment. Specifically, the question was asked if insurance benefits had any effect on the patient's choice of initial provider type, whether the choice of initial provider type had any effect on the costs of care, and whether the insurance benefit had any influence on the costs of care beyond its effect on the choice of initial provider type.

Researchers Ann Holmes, Ph.D., Assistant Professor at the School of Public and Environmental Affairs at Indiana University-Purdue University at Indianapolis, and Partha Deb, Ph.D., Associate Professor in the Department of Economics at Indiana University-Purdue University at Indianapolis (1998), collected data during four personal interviews conducted during 1987 and 1988. Key variables include the type of provider contacted at the beginning of treatment (psychiatrist, other physician, nonmedical mental health care specialist) and the cost for the treatment episode. The method of analysis is as follows. An episode model of demand for mental health care is estimated using a two-step procedure: multinomial probit analysis is first used to determine the factors that influence the choice of initial provider type, right-censored Tobit analysis is used to determine the factors that affect the costs of care, including the type of provider who initiates the care episode.

Essentially the study involves estimating two relationships. First, the researchers estimated the probability that an individual seeks care from a given provider type. Second, the researchers estimated the effect of the explanatory variables on the total costs of treatment, conditioned on decisions made at the first stage.

Results indicate that out-of-pocket costs significantly affect the patient's initial choice of provider type but that, after controlling for provider choice, price is no longer significant in explaining overall treatment costs. After controlling for selection effects, care episodes initiated by nonspecialist physicians are found to be as expensive as those initiated by nonphysicians. Essentially the results conclude that nonmedical mental health care specialists may be more effective than physicians in controlling costs when used as case managers in the care of persons with mental illnesses. Perceived mental health status affects the choice of initial provider type: people who feel anxious are more likely to seek care from a physician, whereas those who feel depressed are more likely to seek care from nonphysician specialists. The price of psychiatrist visits has no statistically significant effect on the choice of initial physician type. Thus, patients are more likely to seek care from a nonphysician than from either type of physician if the expected out-of-pocket costs are lower for nonphysician care. These estimates indicate that changes in insurance benefits can influence initial provider choice.

It is important to point out that policy would be badly misguided by cost estimates that do not correct for patient selection and other factors, since such uncorrected estimates suggest that nonphysician providers are relatively more expensive than physician providers. Insurance benefits should not only include the services of nonphysician providers, but should be designed to encourage their use.

3.5   COMPETITION VERSUS REGULATION: WHAT APPROACH IS MORE EFFECTIVE?

The problem explored in the paper is: Should Americans rely on market forces or on government regulation to contain spiraling health care costs?

The study included analysis of the statistical data related to the hospital discharge costs in 15 States with the highest HMO penetration. The goal was to determine the effectiveness of market-based strategies in controlling the health care costs and to provide guidance to the State regulators in establishing health care policies.

The researcher, Thomas P. Weil (1996), is President of Bedford Health Associates, Inc., a health care management consulting firm in Asheville, North Carolina. The published health care statistics as well as data acquired via personal communications, were used in determining the HMO penetration rates in individual States and in calculating the adjusted hospital discharge rates.

To compare States with different economic and demographic conditions, the hospital discharge rates were adjusted for case mix severity and the Medicare wage index. Further adjustments were made for the medical education-type expenses (number of residents in approved training programs per 100,000 persons), and for the use rates (annual number of patient days per 1,000 persons).

It was found that a higher HMO market penetration does not per se result in lower hospital costs. It was found that either relative inefficiency of the State-managed hospital reimbursement rates (New York, Massachusetts), or a high discharge rate (Missouri) can contribute to high per-capita hospital care cost. Annual growth of reimbursement rates was much higher than the annual inflation rate in all of the States, suggesting need for cost containment measures.

It was found that the annual pre-capita hospital cost is strongly tied to the number of paid employee-hours per adjusted discharge for either a "highly regulated" or a "highly competitive" State. Minimizing business expenses and centralizing sophisticated services helped to minimize the average per-capita hospital cost in all types of business environments (regulated, market-driven, and mixed).

The researcher argues that installing spending caps such as capitation fees for HMOs or Medicare reimbursement rates by the government can lead to similar cost reductions, but in different ways. This is a highly political issue, with each approach having its advocates and its critics. The market-driven approach usually adds barriers to accessibility of services, while the statutory approach often adds difficulties to setting eligibility for benefits, causes inequities among providers and adds inefficiencies. Growth of the powerful provider networks and their associated HMOs, especially in metropolitan areas, raises concerns for potential monopolization of the health care system.

The researcher advocates blending of the two approaches and decentralization of the regulatory efforts to the State/local level to maximize ability of the States to match available resources to local health care delivery needs. Based on statistical data studied, he argues that such a blending is already occurring in a number of States, such as New York and Maryland, with high penetration of HMOs and also with reimbursement rates being aggressively regulated by the State agencies. Which shape this blending will eventually take under the competing political forces remains to be seen.

3.6 THE COST OF OBESITY IN THE UNITED STATES

Medical costs in the United States are escalating at an alarming rate. Many studies have been undertaken to dissect these costs, in the hope of finding remedies. Managed care efforts to control the problem have yet to come up with long term solutions. Despite the fact that Americans spend billions of dollars each year on ways of improving their health, obesity continues to plague a large percentage of the population. This study attempts to estimate the direct and indirect costs of obesity-associated disease in the US in 1990.

Researchers A. M. Wolf and G. A. Colditz (1994) of the Harvard Medical School Channing Laboratory estimated the economic costs of obesity-associated diabetes, cardiovascular disease, gallbladder disease, cancer, and musculoskeletal disorders in 1990 US dollars, using a prevalence-based approach to cost-of-illness. They also calculated indirect costs by calculating work days lost, and calculated mortality costs based on lifetime earnings lost.

To determine the 1990 economic costs of non-insulin-dependent diabetes mellitus (NIDDM), the researchers utilized the 1980 published estimates of US healthcare expenditures (Hodgson & Kopstein, 1984). These costs included routine care for NIDDM, costs related to morbidity and mortality from NIDDM complications, and costs resulting from the prevalence of other diseases due to uncontrolled NIDDM. Costs were increased in proportion to the increase in population and per capita healthcare expenditures. Total direct costs of NIDDM were estimated to be $15.5 billion. Based on statistics from the Nurses' Health Study and others, the researchers estimated that 57 percent of these total costs, or $8.8 billion, are attributed to obesity.

The ongoing Nurses' Health Study estimates that 90 percent of the gall-bladder disease cases in the US are directly attributable to obesity. The researchers therefore calculated the economic cost of gallbladder disease attributable to obesity as $3.2 billion.

Based on study data (Colditz, 1992 and Manson, et al., 1990), the researchers assumed that 27 percent of cardiovascular disease is diagnosed among the obese, and that among the obese 70 percent of the disease is directly attributable to obesity. Economic costs of cardio-vascular disease attributable to obesity were therefore estimated to be $29.4 billion.

Based on study data linking cancer to increased weight (Lew & Garfinkel, 1979) and other perspective data, the researchers concluded that 2.3 percent of the total costs of cancer should be attributed to obesity. Therefore, the direct cost of obesity related cancer was estimated to be $0.68 billion.

In a similar fashion, it was estimated that 10 percent or $3.75 billion of the economic costs of musculoskeletal disease was attributable to obesity.

Indirect costs represented the costs of lost output caused by morbidity and mortality due to obesity. Using 1988 National Health Interview Survey data and 1989 Handbook of Labor Statistics, the researchers multiplied the marginal number of work days lost due to obesity by the number of obese individuals and the gender- and age-specific daily wage statistics. This calculation resulted in $4 billion in lost work days being attributed to obesity. Indirect costs from mortality due to disease associated with obesity were estimated to be $18.9 billion.

Based on these analyses, the researchers estimated the total direct and indirect costs of obesity in the US in 1990 to be $68.8 billion. While admitting that the accuracy of many of their estimates is questionable, the researchers consider these estimates to be, if anything, conservative.

According to the researchers, obesity represents a *modifiable* contributor to healthcare costs in the US. They stress the importance of programs designed to prevent weight gain and to educate the public on the medical hazards of obesity. With the rate of obesity increasing in recent years the reported estimated costs of obesity will rise substantially in the future. The eye-opening data presented here should impact the decision processes of US government and managed care providers alike.

3.7   COST AND FINANCING OF CARE FOR HIV DISEASE PATIENTS

The treatment of the human immunodeficiency virus (HIV) disease has been transformed by the rapid growth in the number of drugs approved to treat it. Used in combinations of three, the protease inhibitors and antiretroviral drugs are components of the new drug treatment known as "drug cocktails." This is now the regimen of choice and since late 1995, when the cocktail became available, the death rate attributable to acquired immuno-deficiency syndrome (AIDS) has decreased significantly. The infection rate, however, remains the same. The most recent estimate by the Center for Disease Control and Prevention (CDC) in 1996 of the number of people living with HIV disease in the US was 650,000-900,000. The CDC estimated 259,000 AIDS cases in early 1997. While the drug cocktail promises a longer life with better quality, this new treatment also brings with it significant added costs. Not only are the new regimens more expensive than their predecessors, but as people live longer, they consume more health care resources, further driving up the overall costs associated with HIV disease.

Only two studies have examined costs since the emergence of the new drug cocktails, and there are no recent studies of the insurance status of those with HIV disease. This exploratory study was done by Fred J. Hellinger (1998) of the Agency for Health Care Policy and Research (AHCPR). In the study, he examined the relationship between advances in care and costs, the relationship between race, gender, injection drug abuse and costs, and the financing of care for people with HIV disease. Much of this was a secondary analysis, based on data obtained from various sources, including state and federal agencies, along with other cited studies, too numerous to name in this research.

Advances in Care and Costs

The proportion of costs attributable to hospitalization has fallen, as the portion of costs from drug therapy has increased. For example, in New York, costs from hospitalization fell 21 percent from 1988-1994, while drug costs increased 11 percent in the same period. Monthly costs of treatment for 1994-1995 in various States, before the use of the drug cocktail for a certain stage of AIDS, were estimated at $2,100 - $2,500, with drugs accounting for 16-21% of total costs. Costs from 1996, since the drug cocktail, have been estimated at $3,200 - $4,000, with drugs consuming approximately 25% of those costs.

Relationship between Gender, Race, Injection Drug Abuse, and Costs

Females and Whites were found to be less costly to treat, than males and non-Whites, primarily due to the tendency of males and non-Whites to spend more days in the hospital. The relationship between injectable drug abuse and cost of care was ambiguous.

Financing of Health Care for People with HIV Disease

Costs estimated in this section were not discounted and represented the average payments received by providers. Results indicated an increase in the proportion of people with HIV disease with public insurance and a shift of those covered by Medicaid into managed care plans. A small number of States were found to have monthly capitated rates for those with HIV disease, ranging from $1,000 - $3,000. Not all of these included payment for the drug cocktail. Payment rates varied according to region, with Western states generally paying less than those in the East. People with public insurance were shown to have poorer access to care.

Business Implications

Cumulative costs of HIV disease treatment will continue to rise in the near future. Payment rates need to be based on accurate and current cost data. This data, however, remains fragmented. More information is needed regarding the relationships between costs and the characteristics of patients, providers, and facilities. Comprehensive, accurate data will enable managed care organizations to have appropriate payment rates.

3.8   THE FUTURE LOOKS GOOD FOR PRIMARY CARE: FINANCIALLY SPEAKING

Market forces are changing the face of medicine. By focusing efforts on the "gatekeeper"—the primary care physician, managed care has limited the patient's access to specialty care while reducing overall payments to all physicians. The gatekeeper has become the center of all health decisions. The perceived imbalance (nearly 70% of US physicians are specialists) which blamed specialists for driving up the costs of health care has shifted the focus and the payments to the pockets of primary care. With Medicare reducing specialty residency slots and shifting dollars to primary care, future graduates are altering their focus and questioning the benefits of specialty training.

Managed care has made inroads into high costs. Their strategies have addressed inpatient costs, reduced overall payments to physicians, shifted purchasing responsibilities to payers from patients, limited access to care, and monitored utilization and treatment patterns. The early push by managed care for primary care physicians to take on more responsibilities had some resistance from the medical field. The incremental growth of salaries has lessened this resistance. The introduction of "risk-sharing" has also contributed to the decline in incomes for specialists. Primary doctors have money withheld, usually 10%, in pools—if they meet certain criteria or costs for hospital or specialty care, the withhold is returned to the doctor—the more they send their patients to specialists, the lower their return from the risk pool.

Researchers Simon, Dranove, and White (1998), used data from the American Medical Association's (AMA) Socioeconomic Monitoring System (SMS) to evaluate managed care penetration and the changes in physician income. The SMS database receives 4000 annual responses from physicians and data was used from years 1985, 1986, 1993, and 1994. Physicians were split into three groups

1. Primary Care—general and family practice, internal medicine, and pediatrics,
2. Subspecialists—surgical or internal medicine specialty (cardiologists, orthopedics), and
3. RAPs—radiologists, anesthesiologists, and pathologists.

A multi-equation empirical model was used in conjunction with two-stage least squares. Data was adjusted for States and levels of managed care growth.

The results shows that for a one percentage point increase in managed care penetration, primary care gained $2,263 in real income (subspecialty care gained $530 and RAP lost $1,993). In the period of the study managed care rose 15.2% which translated to the $34,405 increase in income for primary care physicians, $8,062 for subspecialists, and a drop of $30,289 for RAPs. This confirms previous studies that show that managed care is most effective at reducing utilization of inpatient hospital services. RAP physicians are mostly hospital-based and rely on referrals for their services. Previous studies have shown that the reversal of income has only come in the early 1990s.

The study found a significant increase in the incomes of primary care physicians in States with high-managed care growth. The income of the hospital-based specialist was inversely correlated with managed care. The results suggest that the promotion of primary care physicians by HMOs has changed the financial potential of physicians. Newer physician graduates who were previously attracted to high-income specialties now can choose primary care as an option and will not be penalized financially for their choice. The emphasis on primary care physicians by managed care organizations will help lower the costs of providing health care. Increases in elderly populations were associated with higher incomes in all groups since elderly patients require less preventative medical care and more specialized hospital care. Increased wealth in a population increased income for specialists. The future for managed care was positively associated with intermediate firm size and negatively with small and large firms.

The implications for future policy decisions are significant. Federal funding for residency programs can alter the balance of health care spending and the incomes of future physicians. The choice of residencies will also affect teaching hospitals that rely on residency funds to cover their costs. The impact of International Medical Graduates (IMG) on all residency slots is not known at this time but these physicians can fill current openings in specialty training. The change in physician income by managed care has alleviated the role of Congress to pass laws and quota for residency slots. The decreased income for specialists may force them to participate with multiple managed care plans to generate patient volume and income. These specialists and RAPs may also be very receptive to capitated contracts from HMOs to stabilize their income stream. Further growth in managed care to mature market structures will reduce incomes for all physicians. Managed care savings will level off unless they begin to target the middle-sized firm. Selective contracting can enhance savings.

REFERENCES

Bills, D. B. (1987). Costs, commitment, and rewards: factors influencing the design and implementation of internal labor market. *Administrative Science Quarterly,* 32, 1987, 202-221.

Hellinger, F. J. (1998). Costs and financing of care for persons with HIV disease: An overview. *Health Care Financing Review,* 19(3), 5-18.

Hirsch, B. T., & Schumacher, E. J. (1995). Monopsony power and relative wages in the labor market for nurses. *Journal of Health Economics,* 14(4), 443-476.

Holmes, A. M., & Deb, P. (1998). Provider choice and use of mental health care: implications for gatekeeper models. *Health Services Research,* 33(5), 1263-1284.

Huse, D. M., Russell, M. W., Drowns, S., Snydman, D. R., & Hartz, S. C. (1998). Economic impact of piperacillin/tazobactam in the treatment of suspected polymicrobial infections. *Journal of Clinical Outcomes Management,* 5(1), 20-30.

Simon, C. J., Dranove, D., & White, W. D. (1998). The effect of managed care on the incomes of primary care and specialty physicians. *Health Services Research,* 33(3, Part 1), 549-569.

Weil, T. P., (1996). Competition versus regulation: Constraining Hospital discharge costs. *Journal of Health Care Finance,* 22(3), 62-74.

Wolf, M. & Colditz, G. A. (1994). The cost of obesity: The US perspective. *PharmaEconomics,* 5(1), 34-37.

CHAPTER 4

HEALTH CARE COSTS, EFFECTIVENESS, AND QUALITY ISSUES

This chapter addresses the implications of financial costs, cost-effectiveness, and cost-quality issues on health care.

The first four research studies address hospital-related cost issues, and the remaining six studies address such areas as home care, emergency medicine, AIDS services, occupational stress and social support, nursing home ownership, and prospective reimbursement in nursing homes.

The first study addressed hospital administrative costs in hospitals. The study found that hospital administrative costs account for close to 25% of total hospital costs in the USA while these costs in Canada are as low as 9%. Also increases in managed care have not lowered these high administrative costs in the USA.

The second study addressed the benefits of hospital contract management as opposed to managers as hospital employees. The results showed that contract managers had a greater tendency toward cost-minimizing

Proven Solutions for Improving Health and Lowering Health Care Costs, pages 47–65.
Copyright © 2003 by Information Age Publishing, Inc.
All rights of reproduction in any form reserved.
ISBN: 1-59311-000-6 (paper), 1-59311-001-4 (cloth)

behavior than hospital employee managers. The study did not address effectiveness or quality of care.

The third study studied the costs and benefits of decreasing in-patient length of stay of children and adolescents with mental disorders. Two strategies were studied and both were cost effective. In addition both strategies provide personal benefits to the children and adolescents.

The fourth study used a prediction model for hospital closure based on several financial ratios. The model had an overall predictive accuracy of 75% for one to two years prior to actual closure.

The fifth study looked at cost-effectiveness of VA Hospital-based home care for terminally ill patients. The results indicated a significantly lower cost per patient day but also significantly more patient satisfaction.

The sixth study addressed the questions related to the variability among the triage, nursing, and physician acuity assessments in emergency rooms. The researchers found a significant variation between triage, nurses, and physicians in emergency room assessments, thus generating poorer quality of care and higher costs. Measures to improve the emergency room procedures could produce lower costs and improved effectiveness.

The seventh study looked at the AIDS costs and service utilization for pediatric patients. Although numerous demographic results were tabulated, the most important ones are that pediatric AIDS patients are overwhelmingly from economically disadvantaged families, Medicaid was utilized by 92% of the cases, and 58% had household incomes less than $10,000 annually.

The eighth study looked at occupational stress, social support, and the cost of health care. The study found that stress and strain were positively related to health care costs. But the more social support an individual has the lower will be the individual's health care cost. The study also found that lower levels of stress did not affect health care costs.

The ninth study evaluated the effects of ownership and costs in the nursing home industry using data from the State of Michigan. The study found that patient cost was not affected by ownership changes in nursing homes.

The tenth and final study addressed prospective reimbursement and nursing home costs in the State of Maine. The prospective reimbursement system was implemented during the 1980s to lower costs. The researchers found that the prospective reimbursement system actually increased the cost of Medicaid nursing home expenses in the State of Maine, thus opening up the policy question on prospective reimbursement for Medicaid nursing home patients.

In this chapter we have addressed a number of health care costs, cost-effectiveness, and health care quality issues. The results indicate that this comprehensive area needs continuous study to assist decision makers and policy analysts to arrive at decisions that produce optimal outcomes.

4.1 THE PROBLEM OF HIGH ADMINISTRATIVE HOSPITAL COSTS

It has been contended that managed care has helped to lower hospital administrative costs. Such contentions could not be confirmed, as no study had been able to answer the question of how much it cost to administer America's hospitals. Previous studies had only been based on data for the State of California. It was therefore not possible to make conclusions for the entire United States.

Researchers Steffie Woolhandler, David U. Hummelstein, and James P. Lewontin (1995) of the Center for National Health Program Studies examined the expenses of 6,400 hospitals in the United States. Their research was in search of answering the question of how much it cost to administer America's hospitals.

The researchers based their analysis on the Medicare Cost Report. The report was provided to them by the Health Care Financing Administration. The authors had to subjectively determine which costs reported to Medicare were administrative, and which were not. The researchers determined that the administrative and general costs including nursing administration, central services and supply, medical records and library, skilled nursing facility, utilization review, and salary costs of the employee benefits department cost categories should be considered administrative.

The Medicare Cost Report did not allocate the hospital's physical plant to the individual hospital functions. As a result, the researchers had to assume that administration's share of physical plant costs would be the same as its share of overall costs. As stated above, the authors classified all of the salary costs of the employee benefits department as administrative. All other employee benefit costs were allocated to administrative costs based on administration's overall share of costs.

To determine administration's proportion of total costs, the researchers added all of the administrative costs, the allocated shares of physical plant and the allocated shares of employee benefits, and divided the sum by total hospital costs. The authors also determined each State's average amount of costs devoted to administration.

The researchers discovered that an average of 24.8% of total fiscal 1990 hospital costs were administrative. They also found that administrative salaries were an average of 22.4% of total hospital salaries. The authors also discovered that States with larger managed care penetration had higher administrative costs as a proportion of total costs. In States where more than 25% of the population belonged to a health maintenance organization, administrative costs were 25.6% of total costs, while administrative salaries were 22.6% of total salaries. On the other hand, in States with less than 25% of the population enrolled in health maintenance organizations, administrative costs were 24.6% of total costs, and administrative salaries were 23.3% of total salaries.

The results are quite interesting. Recent reforms, such as managed care and competitive bidding, have been aimed at trimming hospital administration. However, the results of this study confirm that hospital administrative costs have not declined. This study even found that States with larger managed care populations have higher administrative costs. Canadian hospitals have shown that it is indeed possible for administrative costs to account for as little as 9% of total hospital costs. It remains for America's health care managers to find ways to lower administrative costs to levels similar to those in Canada.

4.2   DOES CONTRACT MANAGEMENT REDUCE COSTS?

A finance theory called expense preference theory states that managers of firms in which ownership is segregated from control (top management does not own the firm) will not minimize cost all of the time. The managers of these institutions are utility maximizers who will spend moneys beyond the cost minimizing amount on salaries, goods, and services (inputs) that they prefer. Within the healthcare industry this theory is rarely examined with respect to hospitals due to the fact that the majority of the institutions are non-profit and are rarely owned and managed by the same people. However, contract-managed hospitals may be tested to determine if contract managers employed cost minimizing inputs and practices.

Avi Dor, Sarah Duffy, and Herbert Wong (1997) test whether hospitals that became contract managed between 1984-1990 had previously employed management who did not minimize costs. It was hypothesized that the contract managers would have incentives to utilize cost minimizing measures (not to display expense preference behavior) because their main function is to improve the financial performance of the institution and renewal of the contract is dependent upon that factor.

The group began by conducting a comprehensive literature search and review for selection of a process to determine expense preference. Previous expense preference research separates firms into two groups, cost minimizers and expense preferencers, through the use of a dummy variable method. However, the researchers decided against this traditional method. They preferred an alternative test in which expense preference is measured by another statistical method.

The researchers developed a mathematical test for expense preference and then preceded to choose hospitals based on the following criterion—the hospital must have opted for contract management during the time frame from 1984-1990. This criterion resulted in a final sample of 189 hospitals. The researchers then tested expense preference separately for the pre-contract and post-contract (using the second year post-contract) period and compared the two periods.

The conclusion of the group was that within health care markets there was evidence suggesting that switching from conventional management compensation to a contract management arrangement reduced the incentives for expense preference behavior. However, it was also discovered that expense preference behavior depends upon the discretionary input being measured and failure to recognize the different types of inputs as related to managerial preferences may cause an underestimation of expense preferencing in other industries.

The conclusion that contract managers did not show a tendency towards expense preferencing has two key impacts within healthcare. The first is that there is now an option available to those healthcare institutions which are experiencing financial difficulty. Previously the only option available to those institutions who were financially unstable was to merge with a financially secure institution and attempt to reduce costs through exploitation of synergies. This research indicates that hospitals experiencing financial difficulty may now opt for a contract manager who has a strong incentive to minimize expenditures.

The second impact is that of managed care. Managed care in some manner tends to force institutions to maximize their resources while minimizing their costs. Hospitals that are having difficulties surviving within the parameters of managed care may consider replacing current management with a contracted team to meet the expectations of managed care and eliminate any expense preferencing that may currently exist.

4.3   COSTS AND BENEFITS OF DECREASING LENGTH OF STAY: TWO STRATEGIES

Health policy makers are challenged by the inpatient care of children and adolescents with mental health disorders. This is because inpatient care, which is the most expensive type of care available, consumes a large portion of the mental health agency's budget (National Health Institute of Mental Health 1987); and due to its availability, is utilized when less restrictive therapeutic environments would be more appropriate. To reduce the amount of time spent in the hospital, preventive services could be provided that would reduce the need for hospitalization or factors that contribute to the excessive stay could be altered.

The researchers Margolis and Petti (1994) analyzed the costs of the two strategies to reduce the length of stay: preventive home-based, family-oriented services, and increased reimbursement for out-of-home treatment. The data source for this study was collected on all children discharged (261) from the state psychiatric hospital (the Hawthorn Center) in Wayne County, Michigan, from 1987 through 1989. Statistical analysis was used to arrive at a sample of 22 children to be used for simulation analysis. The sample of 22 children provided a representation of the larger sample of the 261 children.

The simulation analysis compared the cost of home-based services to the costs of increased payment for community-based placements. The cost of home-based services was estimated to be $3,155 per client (based on the Tacoma-based Homebuilders study) in 1990 dollars. The cost of excessive length of stay was calculated as follows. The per diem cost of hospitalization was arrived at by dividing the total cost of hospitalization by the length of stay. The excessive length of stay (XLOS) was calculated by subtracting the cost of placement per day (obtained from the Hawthorn Center Department of Social Services) from the cost of hospitalization per day. This figure was then multiplied by the XLOS days. The cost of increased out-of-home placement was calculated by multiplying the average stay in out-of-home placements by the number of children placed per year to arrive at the number of beds utilized and then converting this figure to a daily cost.

Remuneration was measured via elasticity—the economic measure of the expected increase anticipated in supply as a result of an increase in price of the commodity. In this case, the expected increase in supply of rooms anticipated as a result of the increase in remuneration. Elasticity was measured to be 1.5 which means that for every one percent increase in payment, there will be a 1.5 percent increase in supply.

The 18 children (76%) targeted for home based services generated a total cost of $56,790. The remaining 24% (4 children) generated a total XLOS cost of $88,707. The XLOS costs could be avoided for 14 of the children, thus saving $310,473 (XLOS rate of $113.61 x 195.2 mean days x 14 children). The overall conclusion of the results is that for every dollar spent on family intervention, $2.12 in XLOS costs could be avoided.

Family intervention is more cost effective than increasing remuneration for out-of-home placement. Intensive home-based services can reduce the need for hospital stay and therefore reduce excessive stays. Also, increased compensation for out-of-home services will increase the supply of community placements and expedite hospital discharge. Although this is not as cost effective as home-based services, it does not add new costs to the mental health system.

The benefit measured in this study was the avoided cost of hospitalization and not the effectiveness of treatment. The emotional and physical costs on families and lost income from staying at home instead of working were also not considered. Increasing remuneration could attract individuals who otherwise would not have the financial means to provide these services. It could also attract entrepreneurs who may be more concerned with earning a profit than with the welfare of the children.

Home-based services provide an opportunity for economic benefit which remuneration does not afford. However, both strategies provide personal benefits to those children affected. Home care minimizes the stigma associated with hospitalization and increased remuneration encourages patients to assume more responsibility for their selves. Both strategies deserve consideration for further implementation and they both offer to provide care in the "least restrictive" environment.

4.4 PREDICTION MODEL FOR HOSPITAL CLOSURE USING ACCOUNTING DATA

Health Care Delivery has increased steadily in competition since 1970. The increase of costs and the decrease of reimbursements forced many hospitals to close. It was estimated at the time of this study that 700 U.S. hospitals would close between 1987 and 1995. Many financial studies have been used to predict corporate bankruptcy. Prediction models for corporate bankruptcy do not fit all economic sectors, particularly the service sector. Research that had been done for hospital closure did not address financial predictors and did not use a set of closed hospital data.

Paul Wertheim of the Business Administration Division at Pepperdine University, Malibu, California, and Monty L. Lynn of the Department of Management Sciences at Abilene Christian University, Abilene, Texas (1993), sought to identify financial variables as vital predictors of hospital closure. They utilized 21 financial ratios under the four broad categories of leverage, liquidity, capital efficiency, and resource availability. The tested hypotheses are shown below.

- Closed hospitals will tend to have a higher leverage ratio than open hospitals for one year or two years prior to closure.
- Closed hospitals will tend to have a lower liquidity ratio than open hospitals for one year or two years prior to closure.
- Closed hospitals will tend to have a lower capital efficiency ratio than open hospitals for one year or two years prior to closure.
- Closed hospitals will tend to have a lower asset availability ratio than open hospitals for one year or two years prior to closure.

Statistical models were used to predict hospital closure using matched data from closed and open hospitals. Cost reports from Health Care Financing Administration and the Annual Medicare Hospital Cost Report were utilized. Hospital closure for this study was measured as the "Permanent closing of a hospital facility and the discontinuance of the provision of inpatient medical care, whether acute or chronic."

As a prerequisite to be selected for the final sample of closed hospitals, financial data two years prior to closure was required. The sample selected consisted of 71 hospitals that closed anywhere from 1983 to 1987. Selected to be matched to the closed set were 71 open hospitals with two years of financial data from 1983 to 1987. Three factors that were used for matching open hospitals were:

1.   Geographical location,
2.   Urban versus rural status, and
3.   Number of beds.

Matching began with the closed hospitals and then an open hospital was randomly chosen that had all three factors in common with the closed hospital.

The twenty-one financial ratios were used as independent variables. Although as many as 34 financial ratios have been used in previous studies to predict bankruptcy, not all are useful in hospital closure and for some, data was not available. Time intervals of one and two years prior to closure are used.

One and two years prior to closure "closed" hospitals showed higher debt ratios and lower liquidity, capital efficiency, and asset availability ratios than "open" hospitals. The one year prior to hospital closure study results show that 17 out of 21 ratios are significantly related to hospital closure. The best predictor was the ratio of net income/total revenues, the profitability ratio. This variable was 70.6% accurate at predicting closed hospitals. Predictive results for two years prior to closure were weaker with only 8 or the 21 ratios statistically significant in the prediction model.

A multivariate model gave additional explanatory power to predict hospital closure. To keep the model simple, one ratio from each of the four categories (leverage, liquidity, capital efficiency, and resource availability) was chosen. This multivariate model had the highest values for sensitivity (78.3%), and overall predictive accuracy.

Both univariate and multivariate models are useful predictions for one and two years prior to hospital closing. Both models are accurate and simple. Hospitals can use these financial indicators to detect problems early on, develop appropriate financial tactics earlier and choose strategies to enhance performance. Buyers interested in an acquisition or merger will have a better handle of the financial viability of the hospital before acquiring or merging. All stakeholders can benefit by knowing how viable financially his/her particular hospital is.

4.5   COST EFFECTIVENESS OF HOSPITAL-BASED HOME CARE

The high cost of treating patients with terminal illness has gained a lot of attention. Due to increasing costs and issues concerning the appropriateness of care for terminally ill patients several studies have been conducted examining the appropriateness of home care (HOSPIC) compared to acute inpatient hospital care. However, little has been done to examine the cost effectiveness of this care. Therefore, Hughes, Cummings, Weaver, Manhein, Braun, and Conrad (1992) examined the cost effectiveness of home health care in the treatment of the terminally ill.

The researchers hypothesized that home health care would cost less than customary care in the treatment of patients with terminal illness, without harming patients. The study they performed consisted of terminally ill patients (with informal caregivers) who presented themselves for treatment at The Edward Hines Veterans Administration (VA) Hospital. All admissions from April 1984 to May 1987 were screened, from which 171 patients were selected and randomized. Analysis was conducted on both the control group (85) and the home-based health care group (86). The control group of patients were allowed to access customary care within or outside the VA hospital system. While the study group had access to hospital-based home care (HBHC).

Baseline and follow-up interviews (one month, six month) were given to assess the patient's cognitive and functional status as well as to assess the morale and satisfaction with care of both the caregiver and patient. Care given to all patients (ambulatory care, emergency room (ER) visits, etc.) both within the VA system and within the private sector were monitored through the use of patient (caregiver) health care diaries.

The results of the study indicated:

- At the end of one month there were no significant differences in activities of daily living (ADL) or cognitive measures; however, at the end of the first month there was a significant difference in patient satisfaction with the HBHC group being more satisfied than the control group.
- Those receiving HBHC averaged significantly fewer days hospitalized compared to the control group (10 vs. 15.9). On average HBHC patients spent 3.5 fewer days in the hospital prior to death compared to the control group.
- The mean number of clinic visits was significantly higher for the control group (2.59) compared to the HBHC group (.73). However, the number of home nursing visits for the HBHC group was significantly higher than the control group (17.9 vs. 7.1).

In the cost analysis it was determined that the cost of home health care visits was higher in the HBHC group than in the control group; however, these costs were offset by significantly lower hospitalization costs. When net per capita health care costs for the two groups were compared there was a cost savings of $769 per patient seen in the HBHC group. This cost savings indicates that HBHC could be a cost effective means of caring for those terminally ill patients.

The authors concluded that those patients participating in the HBHC group received both continuous and comprehensive care which was regarded highly by both the caregivers and the patients. There was a powerful substitution effect for home health resources rather than inpatient based resources resulting in shorter hospitalizations and lower overall costs. The results of the study, however, could only be viewed as suggestive at this time and further analysis needs to be performed.

This study is significant because currently only Medicare offers a HOSPIC benefit. However, the waiting period of two years (to be considered disabled) is frequently longer the life expectancy of the patient. Health Maintenance Organizations, in their effort to reduce health care costs while promoting quality care may wish to consider offering HOSPIC riders to their participants under the age of 65. These riders, if utilized, would reduce the organization's hospitalization costs while still providing quality care to the patient.

4.6   EFFECTIVENESS OF ADMISSION DIAGNOSIS IN EMERGENCY MEDICINE

As is the case in most service industries, the quality of service (in this case the quality of care) can be closely related to associated costs. How can a health care organization, especially the emergency department of a hospital, reduce costs without compromising care of the patients? To further complicate this problem it becomes difficult in an emergency room setting to determine where the opportunities of improvement lie, and how can they be identified? This study of emergency medicine provides evidence through statistical analysis of existing hospital data that it is possible to identify areas of potential cost reduction (specifically proper utilization of resources) and pursue cost reduction without compromising patient care.

Researchers Timothy D. West and Sharon A. Pitzer (1997) performed a statistical analysis of existing data from a large community teaching hospital. They examined emergency room acuity assessment data for 3,671 patients. In this study the measure of quality is defined as assessment variability and costs (consumed resources). The question asked is how these costs are associated with nursing and physician diagnosis.

Four primary questions were developed by the researchers to help direct this study. These questions related to the variability among the triage, nursing, and physician acuity assessments. In other words, how many times did the diagnosis of the criticality of the patient's need for care differ among triage, nurse, and physician evaluation? These questions also examined how the triage, nursing, and physician's assessments of required diagnostic resource consumption were related. Note that triage is defined as the initial activity of prioritizing patient's need for care usually done by a nurse or emergency medical technician.

The study consisted of three variables: the pretreatment assessment of the acuity variable (triage), the post-treatment nursing acuity assessment codes, and the physician resource based assessment codes. The triage and nursing acuity assessment were also used to predict resource consumption based on the classification given to the patient. The classifications of patients were immediate care (emergent), urgent care, or routine care. The doctor's resource-based assessment was directly related to the amount of time spent with the patient and the various codes used by physicians were collapsed into three categories corresponding to emergent, urgent, and routine care. The researchers' analysis then focused on the level of agreement between the pretreatment and post-treatment assessments.

The results of the statistical analysis allowed the researchers to develop answers for the four questions that they had posed prior to this study. They determined that there was a significant statistical variation among the assessments by triage, nurses, and physicians. The three assessments only matched in 56% of the cases. This means that 44% of the time the diagnostic resources are either being overutilized or underutilized. About 35% of the triage acuity assessments did not agree with the nursing acuity assessments and 81% of these disagreements had triage considering the care to be routine when the nurses actually performed urgent care, using more resources than predicted by triage. The nurses' acuity assessments differed from the doctors' acuity assessments 35% of the time and of these disagreements, 96% had the physician underclassifying the patient as requiring routine care when the nurse classified them as needing urgent or emergent care. Finally the triage and physician assessments were consistent 79% of the time. Overall the percentage of patients considered to require routine care are as follows (by group), triage 75%, nurses 58%, and physicians 88%.

This study shows that there is a significant variation between triage, nurses, and physicians in emergency room assessments. Evaluation of the decision processes in order to benchmark them against each other can be very beneficial in controlling costs and improving quality. Determining the root cause of the variation will allow the emergency room to provide better services to those who need then and to improve the effectiveness of their services. When there is a disagreement in assessments then there is the likelihood that the true needs of the patient are not being met, which is obviously of great concern for those requiring urgent and emergent care. The allocation of diagnostic resources is an important issue in emergency rooms and consistent accurate assessments will improve planning and the ability to meet the needs of patients. Also since labor costs are a significant portion of an emergency room's overhead, overutilization, and underutilization are costly problems that need to be addressed if emergency rooms want to get costs under control. By better aligning the patient's needs with the service provided, the emergency room can reduce costs and improve quality since the patients will get the care they need, when they need it, and can be charged appropriately.

4.7   AIDS COSTS AND SERVICE UTILIZATION FOR PEDIATRIC PATIENTS

What are the effects of demographics on medical usage by pediatric AIDS patients? Do characteristics such as per capita income, functional status, and social severity have an effect on medical care visits among pediatric AIDS patients? Pediatric AIDS is among the top five causes of death among children although pediatric AIDS cases constitute only approximately two percent of total AIDS cases in the United States. No research to date has examined the influence of low socioeconomic status upon health care utilization patterns for pediatric AIDS patients. This study seeks to do so.

The AIDS Cost and Service Utilization Survey (ACSUS) provided the data for the research (Fahs, et al., 1994). This was an 18-month, federally funded survey conducted by the Agency for Health Care Policy and Research. Pediatric patients at seven hospitals in five cities were sampled with the information provided by the person accompanying the child to the hospital visit. This study utilizes the data from the first six months of the ACSUS. The researchers studied various care services provided for pediatric AIDS in an attempt to study the immediate plight of children with AIDS or HIV symptomatic illnesses. They also studied the measures of social and economic factors that influence the use of medical and support services by children with AIDS. The total sample originally consisted of 141 children, but after losing six to follow-up, 135 children were left at the end of the six-month survey period.

The study measured per capita income, functional status, and social severity. Per capita income was measured using total household annualized monthly income estimated based on household size. Functional status was assessed using a series of questions on motor and social development from the National Health Interview Survey conducted by the U.S. Department of Health and Human Services, Public Health Service, National Center for Health Statistics.

Social severity was analyzed using three dimensions of the child's social environment: family structure, economic security, and informal personal network. Family structure consisted of household composition, number of HIV-seropositive persons in the house, and language. There were two options for the family structure: Two parents or kin living in the household or other. There were three options for the number of HIV+ persons in the household: No HIV+ persons, No HIV+ relative or foster parent, or one or more HIV+ relatives or foster parents. Language was defined as either

English or Spanish. Demographic information was also provided on the patient's sex, age, and race.

Economic severity was defined by housing and annual income. Housing was either owned/leased by caregiver or other. Annual income was characterized by three levels: greater than $20,000 excluding public programs, over $20,000 including public programs, or less than $20,000. Informal personal network was defined as help from family and friends as caregivers and was characterized by three levels: 20 hours or more per week, 10-19 hours per week, or less than 10 hours per week.

The demographics of the research found the following. The population was split 52% male and 48% female. Fifty-four percent of the population was 48 months or older, and 79% was 22 months or older. The group surveyed was 62% African-American, 25% Hispanic, and 10% Caucasian which indicates that the African-American and Hispanic populations are over-represented compared to their percentage make-up of the general population. Approximately 92% of the sample spoke English as their primary language. Sixty-one percent of caretakers owned or held lease to their housing, while 37% paid rent. Medicaid was utilized by 92% of the population. Thirty-one percent of the sample had household incomes of less than $5,000 and 58% had incomes of less than $10,000 demonstrating how this low income group is over-represented compared to the general public which represents 15% of those having incomes below $10,000. Almost two thirds of the population received some form of public assistance.

Hospital clinic visits ranged from 1.45 to 45.98 with mean number of visits of 7.34. Approximately half of the sample visited the emergency room during the six-month period with the mean visit at 1.27 per child. Forty children were hospitalized for 614 days or an average of 4.55 days per child. The average length of stay was 16.03 days. Few children received community-based services outside the hospital or outside of mental health services. Functional status did not appear to have an effect on informal home care but did appear to be related to hospital utilization and private physician visits showed more visits by children with higher functional status. The study showed little variation in utilization rates by children with differing social severity.

The pediatric AIDS population is a group that is comprised mostly by children from disadvantaged families and many of the hospitalizations are caused by social rather than medical factors. Of this group, only 42% are involved in clinical trials compared with much higher percentages, such as 80% for pediatric cancer patients, for other illnesses. Children living in poverty are those least likely to be involved in clinical trials. The question becomes how to reach out to the disadvantaged population and improve the health care provided to pediatric AIDS patients. This may be accomplished by increased government funding, outreach programs, increased clinical trial participation, or expanded heath care facilities. However, whatever is done, this group is suffering more as a result of factors that are in the control of their families or caregivers, as opposed to the deadly AIDS disease.

4.8   EFFECTS OF OCCUPATIONAL STRESS AND SOCIAL SUPPORT ON THE COSTS OF HEALTH CARE

Recent research suggests that occupational stress will ultimately lead to failing health and illness. This is because the more stress an individual feels, the lower his/her resistance is to health problems. Social support helps people deal with stressful situations and therefore reduces the effect of stress on his/her health. In 1993, 90% of patients seeking medical attention, had stress-related symptoms, which cost US industries $68 billion per year. Organizational health care costs are projected to be near 10% of GNP in the year 2000.

Michael R. Manning of New Mexico State University, Conrad N. Jackson of Organizational Change Management, and Marcelline R. Fusilier of Northwestern State University (1996) set out to improve upon recent studies that were lacking objective measures of health. In order to do this, patients' medical records were used to assess the gather information on types of illnesses and their associated costs. Three categories of stress-related variables were used in order to formulate three hypotheses. The variables studied included work events, subjective perceptions of strain, and social support. Age, gender, and previous health care costs were controlled. The study was exploratory in nature and predicted health care costs were developed by using regression analysis. The independent variables were stress, strain, social support, and their interactions. The researchers hypothesized that stressors and strains cause illness, which increases the costs of health care and that the amount of social support available negatively affects health care costs.

Participants were taken from two different companies. The first organization was a small manufacturing division of a multinational chemical company, and the second was a large health insurance company. A total of 260 people participated in the study from all hierarchical levels (143 from the health insurance company and 117 from the manufacturing firm). There were 128 managers and 132 individuals with no supervisory experience, with an average age of 36.88 years (ranging from 21 to 64). The health insurance company provided 38 men and 105 women, while 47 men and 70 women were taken from the manufacturing company.

The researchers compiled surveys to obtain the self-report variables, which concentrated on experiences with stressors, strains, and social support. The social support section was scored for perceived number of social supports and satisfaction with the social support available. The participants also indicated which out of thirty stressful job experiences occurred in the previous twelve months. The strain composite index measured eighteen items with a seven-point scale. Job satisfaction was measured with ten items also on a seven-point scale.

To provide a more objective measure of health, health care costs were measured using economic data, which reflects an individual's health and illness. The health care costs that were included for analysis were physician office visits, hospital outpatient and inpatient treatment, prescription drugs, and miscellaneous health care. These costs were obtained for one year prior to the surveys and one year after the surveys.

Results show that there was some degree of correlation between the self-report and health care cost variables, as predicted. Stress and strain were positively related to health care costs, whereas the number of social supports was negatively related to health care costs. Surprisingly, the researchers found that when there was some amount of stress combined with social support, health care costs were lower than for individuals with very low stress. This suggests that moderate levels of stress when combined with social support is good for workers' health.

This research has critical implications for US organizations. The cost of health care in this country is expected to keep rising. Companies need to realize that the level of stress workers feel is positively related to their health care costs and that the amount of social support can help employees cope. It is important for business firms to try and reduce the levels of stress within their organizations. In addition, companies should encourage social relationships at work.

4.9   OWNERSHIP AND COSTS IN NURSING HOME INDUSTRY

Does the type of ownership or change in ownership within the nursing home environment reflect on industry cost structures? Type of ownership, how many nursing homes are paid for, and the services they provide are considered to be important determinants of cost variation within the nursing home industry. The buying, selling, and stability of ownership of these facilities has raised concerns of quality and cost. The purpose of this study is to examine the effects of facility ownership, and ownership changes in reference to these nursing home cost structures.

Julia Shaw Holmes, Ph.D., (1996) is an assistant professor of the School of Work at the University of Iowa. Her research centers on the effects of nursing home industry cost with the type of ownership or ownership change within the nursing home facility. Facility ownership types were defined as chain, proprietary non-chain, freestanding nonprofit, government owned, and hospital-based.

Holmes used administrative data collected from the Michigan Department of Social Services, Medical Services Administration (Medicaid), and the Michigan Department of Public Health. Cost data for 393 Michigan nursing facilities was collected from 1989 audited cost reports, and other pertinent facility characteristics were collected from the 1989 annual Michigan licensing and certification survey.

Ordinary least squares regressions were estimated to examine ownership effects on both dependent variables: per diem patient costs (labor/support, food, utilities, supplies) and per diem plant costs (interest, taxes, tenure factors) for the entire sample, using a series of four variables for ownership. Estimation techniques and separate regressions by ownership type were studied to test for interaction effects using the key variables of changing facility ownership within the last five years, size, payer mix, case mix, and in-state or out-of-state ownership.

Behavioral differences based on patient care costs among nursing home ownership types tended to distinguish government-owned and hospital based facilities from freestanding homes rather than the usual distinction between for-profit and not-for-profit facilities. This suggested that there was a sort of homogeneity among all types of nursing home facilities. Percent Medicaid, case mix, geographic region, quality, or sizes were also not related to per diem plant cost.

The effects of ownership change and new construction behaved in similar ways for all ownership types. While facility sales increased plant costs, they did not result in additional patient care costs spending. These results suggest that there are perverse economic incentives operating in state Medicaid capital reimbursement systems that favor frequent ownership changes in the proprietary sector. The reimbursement methods for capital costs by Medicaid programs may be indirectly subsidizing facility sales without an accompanying increase in expenditures for patient care. Therefore, these reimbursement methods ultimately increase the frequency of facility sales and costs to state Medicaid programs.

State Medicaid programs were originally designed for acute care coverage for the poor and medically needy populations. However, Medicaid has evolved into the primary payer for long-term nursing home care. With total spending of $59.9 billion in 1991, policymakers are looking for ways to contain costs while ensuring patient quality. Because of the way capital costs are reimbursed by state Medicaid programs, the buying and selling of nursing home facilities as real estate investments has been common rather than the promotion of ownership stability. This has subsequently inflated nursing home rates. Therefore, policymakers have moved aggressively towards restructuring their reimbursement methodologies and limit nursing home bed supply. Evidence of how these factors relate to the rising nursing home industry costs can be determined from this research, allowing policymakers to start controlling and containing the substantial financial burdens both the private individuals and public payers carry.

4.10 PROSPECTIVE REIMBURSEMENT AND NURSING HOME COSTS

The need for cost reductions has been a major challenge for the health care industry as well as for any other. This issue is even more apparent in the case of nursing homes, which have faced rising costs for over two decades since the 1960s with a growth rate higher than any other sector in the health care industry in addition to seeing their budgets become smaller and smaller.

One proposed solution is the replacement of retrospective reimbursement systems with prospective payment systems. Under the first system, nursing homes are provided with a target rate, but any cost incurred above that rate is still paid by the State at the end of the year, at least up to a ceiling. Under the latter system, on the other hand, the rates are set in advance, any savings is either kept by the nursing home or shared with the State. Yet, if the actual costs for the year are higher than the rate, the difference has to be absorbed by the nursing home. Earlier research on the effects of these payment systems on costs have resulted with inconsistent and even conflicting results as to which system is more effective.

Researchers Andrew F. Coburn Richard Fortinsky and Catherine McGuire of the University of Southern Maine and Thomas P. McDonald of the University of Kansas (1993) study this issue in Maine, where the prospective reimbursement system has been implemented in 1982 in Medicaid nursing homes. They focus on the following three questions: how effective this new system has been on slowing down the rate growth in costs, how the cost structure has been affected, and how well the nursing homes performed under the new payment system.

The study spans over six years. The last three years before the implementation are compared to the three years after the implementation. A time-series regression model is used to identify the impact of the new system on the nursing home costs, controlling for variables such as facility characteristics, nursing home market factor, facility case mix and quality of care. The dependent variable is the total Medicaid allowable variable costs per patient day composed of nursing, consulting, dietary house keeping laundry, plant operation/maintenance, and administrative costs. These components are also segmented into three categories: namely, the patient care costs including the first two variables plus drugs, the administrative costs, and the room and board costs which include all the remaining variables. The independent policy variables are: the study year variable which takes values from one to six, the dichotomous reimbursement type variable, and an interaction term of those two. The regressions are run twice; first with exclusively the policy variables and then with the controlled variables included. In both the restricted and full models all the policy related variables appear to be significant for both the total variable costs and its components. The only exception is for the full model for administrative costs where the significance of the reimbursement variable is low and the interaction term is insignificant. The results indicate that the implementation of the prospective reimbursement system significantly decreases the growth in costs. One shortcoming of the research is that it does not adequately capture inflationary pressures on cost and therefore it is difficult to separate the growth decrease in costs due to the payment system from that due to the reduced inflation in those years. The study also separates the nursing homes according to whether they produced savings or incurred loses in the first three years after the implementation. Both the decrease in the savings and the increase in the losses in the third year raise the question of whether the ability of the nursing homes to keep the costs below the reimbursement diminishes over time.

As for the analysis of the reallocation of the resources over the six years, there is no significant change. Yet, there is a decrease in the room and board costs. The implication of this result can be that there is either a decrease in the quality of the services or an increase in the efficiency. Another result of the study is that there are no significant changes in the rate of access of Medicaid patients over the years, yet there is an obvious drop in the last year, which is not conclusive in itself, but should be watched cautiously.

The study provides us with some interesting results about how the prospective reimbursement plan affects the growth of the Medicaid nursing home expenses. It certainly provides some policy implications, specifically that the system should be designed very carefully since some elements can act as a disincentive for cost containment, such as the calculation of the target rate in Maine. The target rates in this case are based on the previous year's rate net of the savings to the State. This result acts as a disincentive to reduce costs for the nursing home costs. This research also opens up further discussions on the impact of these plans on the quality of service and ease of access.

REFERENCES

Coburn, A. F., Fortinsky, R., McGuire, C., & McDonald, T. P. (1993). Effect of prospective reimbursement on nursing home costs. *Health Services Research, 28*(1), 45-68.

Dor, A., Duffy, S., & Wong, H. (1997). Expense preference behavior and contract management: Evidence from U.S. hospitals. *Southern Economic Journal, 329*(6), 400-403.

Fahs, M. C., Waite, D., Sesholtz, M., Muller, C., Hintz, E. A., Maffeo, C., Arno, P., & Bennett, C. (1994), Results of the ACSUS for pediatric AIDS patients: Utilization of services, functional status and social severity. *Health Services Research, 29*(5), 549-569.

Holmes, J. S. (1996). The effects of ownership and ownership change on nursing home industry costs. *Health Services Research, 31*(3), 327-347.

Hughes, S. L., Cummings, J., Weaver, F., Manhein, L., Braun, B., & Conrad, K. (1992). A randomized trial of the cost effectiveness of VA hospital-based home care for the terminally ill. *Health Services Research, 26*(6), 801-817.

Manning, M. R., Jackson, C. N., & Fusilier, M. R. (1996). Occupational stress, social support, and the costs of health care. *Academy of Management Journal, 39*(3), 738-750.

Margolis, L. H., & Petti, R. D. (1994). An analysis of the costs and benefits of two strategies to decrease length of stay in children's psychiatric hospitals. *Health Services Research, 29*(2), 155-167.

Wertheim, P., & Lynn, M. L. (1993). Development of a prediction model for hospital closure using financial accounting data. *Decision Sciences, 24*(3), 529-546.

West, T. D., & Pitzer, S. A. (1997). Improving quality while managing costs in emergency medicine. *Journal of Health Care Finance, 24*(1), 17-29.

Woolhandler, S., Hummelstein, D. U., & Lewontin, J. P. (1995). Administrative costs in U.S. hospitals. *The New England Journal of Medicine, 329*(6), 400-403.

CHAPTER 5

HEALTH MARKETING AND PROMOTION

This chapter covers health marketing issues, surveying practices to elicit degree of client satisfaction with health services, advertising and promotion issues, bargaining between pharmacies and insurers, and rural hospital survival issues.

The first study concerns itself with the marketing of health promotion to sedentary employees of organizations and corporations. The study revealed that 70% of the respondents felt a formal exercise program would be beneficial. The two most preferred categories were "types of exercises" and "degree of difficulty." The study revealed that a formal exercise program would be used by many, but not all, employees.

The second study reported on survey results of nearly 200 hospitals to determine the degree of utilization of product line management (PLM). About 35% of respondents indicated they had adopted PLM, and the results of PLM were higher income per hospital bed, higher gross revenue per bed, higher return on equity, and a lower salary to revenue ratio. The results provide a strong argument for the adoption of PLM.

The third study reports on surveys used by employers to determine how satisfied their employees are with the health care providers accessible to the employees through the company-sponsored health insurance pro-

Proven Solutions for Improving Health and Lowering Health Care Costs, pages 67–79.
Copyright © 2003 by Information Age Publishing, Inc.
All rights of reproduction in any form reserved.
ISBN: 1-59311-000-6 (paper), 1-59311-001-4 (cloth)

grams. Over 50% of the employers surveyed reported that they had dropped their health care providers because of employee dissatisfaction. The main issues in employee dissatisfaction were: lack of respect, lack of compassion, slow service, and unfriendliness. All of the above issues can be rectified with proper health care provider training.

The fourth study also addressed satisfaction with health care providers. However, in this study the provider type was narrowed down to physician practices. Again a survey instrument was used. The results show that the key to holding on to patients lies in patient satisfaction, and especially in the doctor listening to the patient.

The fifth study is concerned with hospital patient satisfaction and how the satisfaction affects the patient satisfaction in future hospital visit encounters. The results of the study show that good prior experiences with the health care system had positive effects on the current experiences of the patient with the services provided.

The sixth study addresses the issue of how to obtain the maximum effect per health advertising dollar. The results of the study indicate that the involvement of multiple advertising agencies in the development of an ad draft, and selecting the best ad draft, is much more effective than just using one advertising agency to develop the single ad draft. The optimal number of agencies to use per ad draft is six, and results in a near doubling of effectiveness versus just using one agency to develop and use a single ad draft.

The seventh study focuses on the effect of identifying the most appropriate message for each potential donor in a fund raising campaign. It was found that the extra work involved in identifying what type of message is most appropriate for each target donor is well worth the effort expanded in terms of net returns.

The eighth study explores the area of individual versus chain store pharmacies and their respective marketing power. The results indicate, not surprisingly, that the concentration inherent in chain store pharmacies gives them considerably more bargaining power. To compensate for this, individual pharmacies have wanted to use collective bargaining to improve their insurance revenues. Antitrust law has prohibited this. The paper argues for elimination of this ban to level the playing field for all pharmacies.

The ninth and final study asked if rural hospitals can survive. A survey in a Southwestern state community revealed that the survival of rural hospitals is problematic especially if an urban medical center is within reasonable travelling distance. The urban hospital is nearly always able to provide more comprehensive care including all of the medical specialties usually not found in rural hospitals. Also the younger population generally opted for care in the more comprehensive medical centers despite the added travel costs.

In this chapter we have addressed a number of issues encountered in the health marketing area including marketing of health promotion, product line management, client or patient satisfaction in general, in a medical practice setting and in a hospital setting, development of effective advertising, developing appropriate messages to potential donors, bargaining between pharmacies and insurers, and the survival probability of rural hospitals.

5.1   EXERCISE IN THE WORKPLACE: MARKETING HEALTH PROMOTION

The past few years have seen a virtual explosion in the use of computers in corporate America. As a result, much of the work now done by personnel in all departments is sedentary. Sedentary work involves "constrained postures," which puts "static loads" on the musculoskeletal system. Chronic lower back pain, pain in the shoulders, neck, wrists, and upper extremities may result from such sedentary postures. Workers suffering from chronic musculoskeletal injury have reduced morale and productivity within organizations. It has been shown that physical exercise reduces the incidence of chronic injuries which result from sedentary work. The purpose of this study was to find a way to increase the marketability of exercise programs within the workplace, thus improving worker compliance and health.

Researchers Waikar, Bradshaw, and Tate, all from Southeastern Louisiana University (1997), surveyed 203 employees in 21 Southeast Louisiana businesses. Their research was designed to assess employees' *willingness* toward having exercise programs in the workplace (likelihood of participants), and their *preferences* regarding the characteristics of the exercise program.

Before developing their questionnaire, the researchers first conducted a literature review. Past research has shown that many factors, such as task related, ergonomic, workstation related, psychosocial, and demographic factors are all associated with the type and degree of injury reported by employees engaged in sedentary work. In addition it was found that gender was directly related to upper extremity cumulative trauma disorders—women reported at a higher frequency than men.

Based in large part on the information revealed in their literature, the researchers developed a formal questionnaire, incorporating demographic and personal factors and questions on various musculoskeletal and visual complaints. An example of some categories that were preference rated is: ease of comprehending exercise instructions, degree of difficulty of exercise, degree of privacy when exercising, length of exercise breaks, types of exercises. These categories, and others, were preference rated on an ordinal scale, from most to least important, using a given number only once. Data was then analyzed to determine frequency and percentages of responses reported by participants.

Respondents to the study represented a good cross section of industry and businesses. More females than males completed the study, and were evenly distributed between the ages of twenty and fifty. The overwhelming majority indicated that they do experience pain and discomfort as a result of work (82.8%). When asked if they had a prior medical condition that might contribute to their pain, an overwhelming amount said no (84.7%), indicating that the sedentary work was a causal factor. When asked if they thought a formal exercise program would be beneficial to them, 70% indicated yes, 5% indicated no, and 25% were unsure. The preference categories (mentioned in previous paragraph) were rated, and it was discovered that "types of exercises," and "degree of difficulty," were the two most important; "level of embarrassment of exercise" was found to be the least important.

This study has very notable implications for a wide variety of businesses today. Most businesses have a large portion of their employees engaged in sedentary work. These employees are at high risk for cumulative trauma disorders. Effective managers must find ways to decrease the incidence of such injuries, as they negatively affect worker morale and productivity. It has been shown that exercise programs successfully accomplish this goal. However, in order for such a program to work, workers must participate in it. This paper successfully endeavored to uncover the likelihood for participation in such programs, and what facets of such a program should be emphasized in order to maximize worker participation. Managers in all industries can take advantage of this research in developing exercise programs for their own workplaces.

5.2 WHO IS ADOPTING PRODUCT LINE MANAGEMENT, AND WHY?

The product line management (PLM) concept adopted by many hospitals is positively related to a number of operating hospital performance factors. What is not clear from this study is the cause and the effect. That is, does adoption of the PLM concept improve operating performance, or are hospitals with good operating performance more likely to adopt the PLM concept.

The study was conducted by G. M. Naidu, Arno Kleimenhagen of the University of Wisconsin, Whitewater, and George D. Pillari of Health Care Investment Analysis, Inc. of Baltimore, Maryland (1993).

The information for the study was collected from a sample survey of 529 hospitals. A total of 176 completed surveys were returned for a 34 percent response rate. Of the respondents, about 35 percent indicated that they were implementing the PLM concept. The PLM implementers showed a higher net income per bed, a higher gross revenue per bed, a higher return on equity, and a lower salary to revenue ratio. PLM implementers were typically medium-size hospitals located in highly competitive markets serving at least medium-size cities.

The result of the study indicate that the PLM concept is adopted by hospitals in highly competitive markets in medium to large urban areas. It is not an approach that is adopted in smaller and less competitive markets.

The results tend to support the notion that PLM is a useful management tool for hospitals. PLM's effect on operations appears to have a favorable impact on profitability.

5.3   CUSTOMER SERVICE AND SATISFACTION

According to a recent article in *Healthcare Financial Management*, more and more companies are using their employees' rating on services performed to determine whether or not to keep their current provider. This, in turn, forces the healthcare providers to pay more attention to their customers and satisfying their needs.

The researchers Zimmerman, Zimmerman, and Lurand (1997) discovered that many companies used customer surveys to keep track of their providers' performance. These surveys were filled out by the employees and turned into the company. The company then analyzed the data and determined the quality of the services that were performed. They also rated the hospitals and physicians involved. The companies listened to what their employees had to say and acted on their employees' best interest. Some healthcare providers were asked to improve their customer service, others were discontinued due to the lack of focus on the quality of care. More than 50 percent of the participants in a recent survey said that they dropped providers due to unacceptable customer service standards.

Many employees had problems with the hospitals and doctors. In the survey, hospitals scored 7.4 out of 10 for customer satisfaction, and physicians scored slightly higher. They were dissatisfied with the lack of respect, lack of compassion, slow service, and unfriendliness.

To try to correct the problems and improve customer service, many hospitals are teaching training programs. They are utilizing focus groups, and ways to cut waiting times among other methods to better their customer service and to increase customer satisfaction.

Many healthcare providers are using more of their resources to better their customer services skills. They realized that if they don't keep their clients satisfied and happy, they can go to someone else.

5.4   PATIENT SATISFACTION:
THE KEY TO A MEDICAL PRACTICE SURVIVAL

Today's healthcare environment is vastly different from years ago. In the past, physicians simply had to practice in a client rich environment and steady business would follow. Patients listened without question to their doctor's directives and usually had little avenue for complaint. However, doctors today do not have nearly as secure a position. Patients are more educated and have more options. Managed care is transforming the world of medicine into a fiercely competitive market. In order for today's doctor to be successful, he must actively seek out new patients, and continually seek out ways to hold on to his old ones. One of the most effective ways to accomplish this mission is by focusing on "patient satisfaction."

Researchers Philip Nitse, of Idaho State University, and Van Rushing, a private practice internist at Cresthaven Internal Medicine, Memphis, TN (1996), collected data from patients of participating physicians in Tennessee. Their research was designed to determine what aspects of patient care (performance areas) the patients deemed important. In addition the researchers intended to determine the level of patient satisfaction in each of the performance areas.

Data for this study was collected by means of a mail questionnaire. Potential respondents were patients selected from a random array of participating physicians. Subjects were informed that physicians would not see individual responses, but would be appraised of overall response patterns. A traditional importance-performance grid was created. Data landing in quadrant one correlated with "Keep up the good work," in quadrant 2 "Concentrate here," in quadrant 3 "Low priority," and in quadrant 4 "Possible overkill." An example of some of the characteristics assessed is: Having a doctor who listens; Having a doctor who can be easily reached in an emergency; Having a clean and comfortable waiting room; Having reasonable fees, etc. When these performance characteristics are plotted on a grid, the reader can easily assess relative importance and performance.

Respondents were separated into two groups: current patients and ex-patients. Several differences between the two groups became evident upon examination of the questionnaire data. Current patients believe that having a doctor that listens to them is important, and they feel they currently have one. For ex-patients, having a doctor who is easily reached is believed to be very important, and is what they believe that they did not have with their previous physicians.

This type of study has enormous implications for both private practice physicians, and provider networks. As previously mentioned, providers must be proactive about holding on to their patients, in this new, highly competitive healthcare market. The key to holding on to patients clearly lies in patient satisfaction, for just as in any business, a satisfied customer will be a repeat customer. The heart of developing an effective customer satisfaction plan, lies in determining what patients want, so that it can be provided. Applying importance-performance analysis to patient satisfaction provides physicians with a tool for uncovering what patients deem important, and how well they (doctors) perform, within their own patient populations. In addition, the results arrived at by the researchers provide us with some valuable information, that can be useful in all medical practices.

5.5 HOW SATISFIED ARE HOSPITAL PATIENTS WITH HEALTH CARE?

Does a good impression of prior health care experience influence subsequent experiences for patients treated in the same or other health care settings? The above was the research question addressed in a study of patients who had recently received medical services from three different hospitals in a Midwestern U.S. setting.

The study was conducted by John Joby of Bentley College (1992). Two hypotheses were tested. Hypothesis one stated that satisfaction with all previous health care experiences influences perceived quality of a hospital, satisfaction with the hospital, and intention to return to the same hospital. Hypothesis two stated that prior impressions of a specific hospital significantly influence quality, satisfaction with and intention to return to the specific hospital.

A questionnaire survey was conducted by asking about 1,500 patients who had recently received medical services from three different hospitals. Of the 1,500 patients, 353 responded with usable responses. The respondents had a mean age of about 50 years, one third were male, 65 percent were married, and 28 percent were college graduates. Hence, the sample was reasonably diversified.

The results of the questionnaire survey revealed that good prior experiences with the health care system, either as a patient or as a relative or friend of the patient, had positive effects on the current experiences of the patient with the health care services received.

The implications of this study are that maintaining a positive impression and a resultant good reputation of the facility will contribute to the impressions patients will have of the health care facility. Also since apparently people view all health care facilities in a community collectively, good or bad impressions left by other facilities will affect the impressions received at a specific health care facility.

5.6   EFFECTIVENESS OF QUALITY VERSUS QUANTITY OF ADVERTISING

The focus of this article centers around the effectiveness of advertising and how managers can get the most out of their advertising budget. The advertising budget could be broken down into two main areas—the creative rendering cost (creation) of the ad, and the amount spend on media presentation. The current trend is for advertising managers to spend most of the budget on media presentation and neglect creative renderings by working with only one advertising agency. Research and empirical evidence in 1972 brought about the Gross model, which predicts that a company would be better off spending more of the budget on the creative rendering aspect of an ad. The authors of this article looked to study the validity of the Gross model in the context of today's firms.

The study was conducted by three researchers, Gina O'Connor, Thomas Willemain, and James MacLachlan (1996), who are associated with the School of Management at Rensselaer Polytechnic Institute. The study was conducted by examining published data on the effectiveness of ads from both the print media and television media. For the print media 566 ads were used from the "Starch Read Most," and for television 188 ads that appeared between 1984 to 1990 were used from "Ad Weeks" data. The researchers measured the effectiveness of these ads by inverting the published data on "Cost per 1000 Retained Impressions" to obtain "Retained Impressions per Media Dollar."

The researchers proposed a model that was parallel to the original Gross model in an effort to determine the optimal number of creative renderings or ad drafts, that will maximize the measure of retained impressions per media dollar. The model which utilized the ad samples mentioned above, also consisted of many variables such as fixed total advertising budget, cost to produce an ad draft, costs of screening the drafts, and the reliability of the screening process.

Original studies conducted by Gross indicate that the more ad drafts created, the more effective the ad will be. However, many corporations will spend most of the advertising budget on the media presentation and usually work with only one agency. When working with only one agency, companies limit their view of the many creative possibilities and thus limit the effectiveness of their ads. Subsequent studies tend to support the Gross model, such as one by Arnold (1987), which found that a 1 percent increase in ad quality had an effect 20 times greater than that of 1 percent increase in media spending.

The researchers found overwhelming evidence in support of the Gross model and even show that the original Gross model underestimated the benefit of using multiple ad drafts. The study found that as the number of ad drafts increases, so does the average effectiveness of the best selected ad. The results showed that for a single draft the retained impressions per dollar is about 57, whereas with two drafts the number rises to 82, and with the average of the best of five drafts, the retained impressions per dollar increases to 124.

A calculation from the study, which took into account all the variables mentioned above shows that producing an ad equals 5 percent of the total ad campaign budget. The optimal number of drafts is 6 and results in 93.4 retained impressions per dollar. A single draft for the same cost yields only 55 retained impressions per dollar.

This study has major implications for advertising managers, as it presents a model to obtain the most for the advertising dollar. However, implementation will be difficult as it requires a company to change their paradigm away from working with one particular advertising agency, which changes the current partnership format as well as opens the company up to the risk of breaches in confidentiality with the agencies. They also have to embrace the fact that much more work needs to be done at the start of the ad campaign through screening the ad drafts.

5.7 IDENTIFYING MAILING CHARACTERISTICS FOR EACH POTENTIAL DONOR

Direct mail campaigns are usually based on two decision variables: characteristics of the mailing, and characteristics of the targets for the mailing. Past research treats each characteristic separately, even though they clearly are expected to interact. This research study focuses on the interaction of both characteristics on the outcome (the net returns) of the mailings.

The study was conducted by Jan Roelf Bult, of the Monitor Company, Cambridge, Massachusetts, and Hiek van der Scheer and Tom Wansbeek of the Economics Faculty, University of Groningen, The Netherlands (1997).

The experiment involved using mailings with different characteristics to different targets, thus taking both characteristics into account. The resultant data was analyzed to identify the proper strategy which produces the highest net returns. The experiment was conducted by a Dutch health care organization, and application of the two-variable strategy produced a higher net return for its fund raising campaign.

Targeting each potential donor with the most appropriate message will improve the net proceeds of a fund raising campaign. The extra efforts involved in identifying what type of message is most appropriate for each target is well worth the effort expanded in terms of net returns.

5.8   BARGAINING OUTCOMES: PHARMACIES AND INSURERS

It has been reported that large, self-insured employers are starting to treat health care providers like any other supplier and are demanding both higher quality and lower reimbursement rates. Insurers have taken a more active role in bargaining with providers, such as pharmacies, over the prices of services. In this changing marketplace, pharmacy trade associations argue that retail pharmacies have been significantly harmed by these new insurer bargaining strategies.

Contracts that result in low pharmacy reimbursement rates, are viewed as "take it or leave it" contracts because there is often no opportunity for price negotiation. As reimbursement rates erode further, many pharmacies are being forced to close or reduce services, which limits access to pharmaceutical services and pharmacist care, which ultimately will increase total health care costs.

Policymakers, in response to this, are being asked to take legislative action to provide relief on exemptions that prohibit independent pharmacies from collectively bargaining with insurers. Although some evidence suggests that insurer bargaining is changing the retail pharmacy industry, it is not clear that all pharmacies have been unsuccessful in bargaining with insurers. Press reports have revealed examples of pharmacies rejecting insurer contracts. Before policymakers provide this legislative relief to the retail pharmacy industry, they need to understand both the extent of pharmacy bargaining power in these negotiations and the circumstances that enhance or diminish this power. There has been little previous research to guide policymakers.

Researchers John Brooks, William Doucette, and Bernard Sorofman, of the College of Pharmacy and Research for Pharmaceutical Outcomes and Policy Research at University of Iowa (1999), aimed this research to fill the information gap by modeling the bargaining power of pharmacies and insurers in price negotiations and investigating the extent to which bargaining power varies with characteristics of the pharmacy, the insurer, and the pharmacy market. They employed the bargaining model originally used by Brooks, Dor, and Wong (BDW), in 1997 and 1998, to describe hospital and insurer bargaining power by applying it to circumstances surrounding the pharmacy and insurer bargaining process.

It has been theorized that asymmetric bargaining power stems from factors exogenous to the bargaining process. BDW's retail version of the model defines bargaining power using three prices: P_H, the most the buyer would be willing to pay for a service in a given market, P_L, the minimum that the seller would be willing to accept for that service in a given market, and P_N, the final negotiated price or bargaining outcome. P_H-P_L is the potential gain from the bargaining model to be divided between the pharmacy and the insurer, and P_N-P_L, the portion of potential gain acquired by the pharmacy. The measure of pharmacy power, Y, is the share of the potential gain that a pharmacy keeps as a result of the bargaining process. If Y equals one, the pharmacy has complete bargaining power and does not discount its price from P_H. If Y equals zero the insurer has complete bargaining power and is able to extract the maximum discount from the pharmacy.

The distinguishing feature of this bargaining model framework is that it controls for a range of alternatives available to each bargainer prior to negotiations. This is crucial in estimating the impact of exogenous factors, Z, such as market structure on bargaining power. The insurer will not pay more than the retail price in a local market, and in the long run the provider cannot charge less than its cost. In other words if retail prices and costs vary across markets, data showing that an insurer paid a lower price in market 1 than in market 2, may not reflect greater insurer power in market 1. Retail prices in market 1 may simply be lower than in market 2.

The data for the study was obtained from the following sources: Medstat's database of 6.8 million pharmacy claims, Sources Informatics' database containing the drug transactions from 35,000 chain and independent retail drug stores nationwide, and National Council of Prescription Drug Program's 1994 pharmacy database.

Z variables included standard measures of market structure (pharmacy ownership concentration, pharmacies per capita, pharmacies per employer, percent independent pharmacies, employee concentration index among employers); socioeconomic characteristics (per capita income, percent on public assistance, percent elderly, percent in poverty, percent rural); pharmacy type (independent, chain, other); and a measure of insurer market presence (total insurer claims in three-digit zip codes divided by a population-based estimate of total prescriptions in that area). State-specific and insurer-specific dummy variables were also included in the analysis.

To investigate whether bargaining power estimates vary with products, four distinct pharmaceutical products were selected: Humulin insulin, Mevacor cholesterol tablets, Dilantin seizure capsules, and Zantac heartburn and ulcer medication.

Estimated regression coefficients were run for each independent variable except the state-level, insurer-level, and product-level dummy variable. A negative estimated regression coefficient means that the related factor is negatively related to pharmacy bargaining power and positively related to insurer bargaining power. It is clear that pharmacy bargaining power varies dramatically with exogenous factors. As a result, the observation of little negotiation between insurers and pharmacies probably means that the insurers are accurately tailoring their initial contract offer to reflect the conditions specifically to each bargain. With this in mind the coefficients for the variables describing market structure generally follow expectations. The fewer pharmacies both per capita and per employer in the market are, the greater the pharmacy bargaining power. Pharmacy bargaining power increases when pharmacy ownership is concentrated in a market at a level approximately greater than the concentration of three or less equivalently sized ownership groups. On the other hand, greater insurer presence in the market, as measured by the percentage of prescriptions in a market that is attributable to the insurer, results in lower pharmacy bargaining power with the insurer. The number of pharmacy employees per capita in a market area is positively related to pharmacy bargaining power.

It should be noted that the qualifications of the data used in this study may limit the generalization and interpretation of the analysis and that the sample used may not be representative of *all* pharmacy and insurer interactions. With this in mind the results support the use of bargaining models when analyzing medical care prices determined by the interaction between pharmacies and insurers with varying degrees of market power over the consumers.

The results demonstrate a clear relationship between pharmacy concentration and pharmacy bargaining power. As pharmacy ownership in an area becomes increasingly concentrated, pharmacy bargaining power increases. These results may underlie the increase in pharmacy mergers as anti-trust law prohibits independents from collectively bargaining with insurers, leaving many independents with few alternatives other than to close or merge with a chain. The implication that is driven home by these results is that unintended consequences of the existing anti-trust law may be to increase concentration in the retail pharmacy industry and to lose the innovative services provided by independent pharmacies. Policymakers need to take another look at the incentives or disincentives being provided by these laws in the interest of the end consumer—the patient.

5.9   CAN RURAL HOSPITALS SURVIVE?

The future of rural hospitals is in grave doubt especially for those rural hospitals located near larger urban areas where more specialized medical care is available. With declining patient loads, declining revenues, and declining surpluses (or increasing deficits), the rural hospitals face an uncertain future. Against this background a telephone survey of potential hospital clients was conducted to gauge their perceptions about being admitted to their local rural hospital or to a larger urban center.

This study was conducted by three researchers, Carl McDaniel and Roger Gates of the University of Texas at Arlington, and Charles W. Lamb, Jr. of Texas Christian University (1992).

The survey consisted of telephone interviews with a sample of residents in a Southwestern state community with a population of about 20,000 people. Questions asked and tabulated consisted of a approximate age, approximate income, and perceptions of the respective qualities of rural and urban hospitals.

The results of the survey indicated that ending up in a local and rural hospital increases with age and decreases with income. Those respondents who would prefer to be treated in urban medical centers were, on average, younger and more affluent than those who said they would prefer to be patients at the local rural hospital. The results confirmed similar studies performed in other communities.

Mentioned most often as unavailable in the local rural hospital were modern diagnostic equipment or labs, dermatologists, allergists, pediatrics, neonatology, neurology, neurosurgery, cardiology, cardiac/thoracic surgery, chemotherapy, radiation therapy, and cancer therapy.

The implications of this study are that the future of the rural hospitals is problematic, especially for those hospitals located in communities not too far distant to urban medical centers. Assuming that younger and more affluent community members are probably better informed, strengthens the question of how much longer many of the rural hospitals can prevail.

REFERENCES

Brooks, J. M., Doucette, W., & Sorofman, B. (1999). Factors affecting bargaining outcomes between pharmacies and insurers. *Health Services Research, 34*(1), 439-451.

Bult, J. R., van der Scheer, H., & Wansbeek, T. (1997). Interaction between target and mailing characteristics in direct marketing, with an application in health care fund raising. *International Journal of Research in Marketing, 14*(4), 301-308.

Joby, J. (1992). Patient Satisfaction: The impact of past experience. *Journal of Health Care Marketing, 12*(3), 56-64.

McDaniel, C., Gates, R., & Lamb, Jr., C. W. (1992). Who leaves the service area? Profiling the hospital outshopper. *Journal of Health Care Marketing, 12*(3), 2-9.

Naidu, G. M., Kleimenhagen, A., & Pillari, G. D. (1993). Is product line management appropriate for your health care facility? *Journal of Health Care Marketing, 13*(3), 6-17.

Nitse, P. S., & Rushing, V. (1996). 'Patient satisfaction' The new area of focus in the physician's office. *Health Marketing Quarterly, 14*(2), 73-84.

O'Connor, G. C., Willemain, T. R., & MacLachlan, J. (1996). The value of competition among agencies in developing ad campaigns: Revisiting gross' model. *Journal of Advertising, 25*(March), 51-63.

Waikar, A., Bradshaw, M. E., & Tate, U. (1997). Improving marketability of exercise programs: Implications for health promotion in the workplace. *Health Marketing Quarterly, 14*(3), 91-106.

Zimmerman, D., Zimmerman, P., & Lurand, C. (1997). Customer service: The new battlefield for market share. *Healthcare Financial Management,* (October), 51-53.

CHAPTER 6

TOTAL QUALITY MANAGEMENT IN HEALTH SYSTEMS

This chapter addresses the topic of total quality management in general and in a few cases specifically in the health care setting.

The first study reports on an investigation on the effects of leadership and staff participation focusing on the extent of clinical involvement in hospital quality improvement efforts. The research revealed that top management leadership, board leadership, and physician participation showed statistically significant positive relationships with clinical involvement in continuous improvement efforts. These results generally agree with other findings in related fields which show that any new initiatives in any organization to be successful must have the open, visible, and emphatic support of the top leadership in the organization.

The second study is a tutorial on service quality. The author looks at service quality resulting from customers' perceptions about the product, customer expectations about the service provided, and how satisfying customer expectations leads to customer satisfaction. In order to satisfy customer expectations two aspects of quality must be satisfied. They are service reliability and process quality. If both of the aspects are provided

Proven Solutions for Improving Health and Lowering Health Care Costs, pages 81–96.
Copyright © 2003 by Information Age Publishing, Inc.
All rights of reproduction in any form reserved.
ISBN: 1-59311-000-6 (paper), 1-59311-001-4 (cloth)

the firm reaches a consistent level of service quality which will make a customer become a potential loyal customer. The really successful firms depend on a cadre of loyal customers to make them grow and prosper.

The third study is entitled service and product quality: a consumer response. This paper is a research study on the automobile industry but it is essentially a study of service quality based on the service an automobile provides to the customer during its lifetime. The researchers found that the satisfaction a customer gets from vehicle servicing is directly correlated with the probability that the customer will be a repeat customer. The automobile's product and service quality aspects are numerous consisting of reliability, durability, styling, image, appearance, and many more. But the only one that is most important to the customer in making future decisions is perceived quality. This is an important lesson to remember when working on quality improvement projects.

The fourth study explores customer-firm relationships, involvement, and customer satisfaction. The study looked at core and peripheral relationships between customers and the supplier, the U.S. Postal Service. The customers were 66 commercial firms. The researchers found that core factors have the strongest direct relationship with overall satisfaction, although peripheral factors are important also but less so than core factors. The implications are that firms should be aware what the core factors are in supplying services to a customer. Attention to these core services is important to generate customer satisfaction.

The fifth study looks at pay levels and product quality. The key result of the research indicated that product quality may be diminished when high salaries to top managers are not matched by commensurately high wages to lower-level employees. Large differences in pay, called pay inequity, can have substantial negative effects on quality. The data on which this study was based covered over half a million employees in the USA and Great Britain. Hence, it is an issue that top management should ponder when attempting to improve quality of products or services and resultant customer satisfaction.

The sixth study assesses the impact of total quality management in 61 hospitals in Western New York. The results of the study revealed that the hospital culture and the implementation of total quality management is positively associated with a greater degree of quality improvement implementation. Translated this means that hospitals which have cultures that can handle change, use teamwork philosophies, and have empowered employees are more likely to receive a higher degree of benefits from quality improvement implementation. Hospital size had no effect. The implication of the above is that success at total quality management implementation depends on how successful a hospital has been in changing its culture to one that is needed for successful implementation of change.

The seventh study is another study with a health care setting, and describes an assessment technique to determine if a hospital is ready for total quality management implementation. The assessment technique is called rapid assessment technology (RAM), and is based on the Malcolm Baldrige National Quality Award Criteria. RAM gathers input from a focus group of internal and external entities, and the input is then categorized into strengths and opportunities for improvement. The benefit of RAM is that it can be quickly administered and the results provide guidance in the much more lengthy total quality management implementation effort.

The eighth and final study poses the question if Total Quality Management (TQM) can improve the bottom line. The study consisted of an evaluation of publicly available financial accounting data for nearly 400 publicly traded firms that won their first quality award between 1983 and 1993. The researchers found that from six years before until three years after winning the award the mean change in operating income was 107% higher than that of the control sample. Hence, results tend to indicate that overall financial performance improves with the implementation of TQM programs.

The eight studies seem to indicate that total quality management efforts, when successfully implemented, provide benefits in terms of better quality, improved customer satisfaction and improved bottom line results.

6.1 IMPORTANCE OF LEADERSHIP IN HOSPITAL QUALITY IMPROVEMENT EFFORTS

Continuous quality improvement (CQI) and total quality management (TQM) approaches are two overlapping efforts to improve quality in general.

This paper reports on an investigation in the effects of leadership and staff participation on the extent of clinical involvement in hospital CQI/ TQM efforts.

Hypotheses were tested using a two-stage modeling approach. Four dimensions of clinical involvement in CQI/TQM were examined: physician participation in formal QI training, physician participation in QI teams, clinical departments with formally organized QA/QI project teams, and clinical conditions and procedures for which quality of care data are used by formally organized QA/QI project teams. Leadership measures included CEO involvement in CQI/TQM, board quality monitoring, board activity in quality improvement, active-staff physician involvement in governance, and physician-at-large involvement in governance. Relevant control variables were included in the analysis.

The researchers Weiner, Shortell, and Alexander (1997) discovered that top management leadership and board leadership showed statistically significant positive relationships with clinical involvement in CQI/TQM efforts. Active staff physicians involved in governance (leadership) also showed statistically significant positive relationships with clinical involvement. However, the physicians-at-large involved in governance had a statistically significant negative relationship with clinical involvement in CQI/TQM efforts.

The results of the study suggest that leadership from top management, the board, and from physician leadership is important in creating clinical involvement in CQI/TQM efforts. These results generally agree with other findings in related fields that any new initiative in an organization to have any chance of success must have the open and visible support from the top leadership consisting of the top management team, the board, and from influential peers. Also the support must be strong, participative and emphatic.

6.2 QUALITY OF SERVICES

The service industry's number one priority is customer satisfaction. When you have negative customer satisfaction, it usually results in negative word-of-mouth between past customers and potential customers, as well as a bad reputation that can be long lasting and drastic. There are ways in which you can improve upon an already good quality approach, or totally overhaul a really bad one. But it is imperative that service companies constantly keep up with, and continually improve, their quality management in order to keep providing services that customers will demand from the service provider instead of from the competition.

Jean Harvey, University of Quebec at Montreal (1998), looks at the service industry from different points of view. He discusses quality as a result of customers' perceptions about the product, customer expectations about the service provided, and how satisfying customer expectations leads to customer satisfaction. He also discusses techniques that a company can use to improve the quality of the service provided in order to get a positive reaction from the customer, and as a result expand their current and potential client base.

First he discusses the aspects of service quality. Quality of service can be categorized into two components: (1) those dimensions that relate to the customers' wants, and (2) those dimensions that pertain to the process that customers have to put themselves through to get those results. The ability of the service provider to deliver the results that customers want time after time, without unexpected problems, is called quality of results or service reliability. Process quality consists of everything that needs to be done to obtain the result (such as a competent workforce, automation, convenience, etc.). He explains how in the service industry in order to ensure optimal quality of service and to retain current, and to solicit new customers, a service provider must have high process quality, which in turn will lead to high quality results.

Finally he discusses the approaches that he feels are necessary to give service-oriented companies an edge in increasing customer satisfaction, and improving the reputation of the company and of the product. These approaches include: Quality Functions Deployment, Blueprinting, Failsafing, Guaranteeing, and Recovering. Those are the generic approaches that he felt companies could use, but he also stresses that service providers must also include some unorthodox approaches to promote their company as trustworthy. He feels that companies must see their service the way that customers do, allowing their customers to see the whole operation, including what's going on in the inside, set high standards for the company and workforce together, and get the customers involved in the business; let them tell you what is right and what is wrong. So he feels that for the service industry to meet rising customer demands, it must not only incorporate general production management ideas, but also ideas that require some risk and vulnerability.

The conclusion is that customers want a lot and it is a company's responsibility to satisfy those wants or risk going out of business. This is difficult in the service industry because it has to be able to satisfy those wants all the time. The business relies solely on fulfilling the full expectations of the customers. If customers' expectations cannot be fulfilled, they will be dissatisfied, and thus will cease to be a customer. A hotel must make sure that a customer's need is satisfied through a good night's sleep or that customer will not return. So in the service industry, companies must remain wary of customers' desires, needs, and wants, and fulfill them constantly, efficiently, and effectively.

This paper is very important to the service industry because it may shed some light on reasons why their business is failing, give them ideas on how to resurrect it, as well as give them ideas on how to become closer to their clientele. In the service industry the business rests solely on having good relationships with customers and the community. In this fast-paced world people demand many things, and they want them as fast as possible. By reading this tutorial, businesses can get some good insight and ideas on how to increase customer satisfaction, and customer relations just by making their business more efficient and providing their customers with just a little extra in terms of the quality of their service and their product.

6.3   SERVICE AND PRODUCT QUALITY: A CONSUMER RESPONSE

When automobile companies look for ways to improve total customer satisfaction, there is more to be looked at than just a solid product. More specifically, the recent loss of market share by American manufacturers to Japanese imports is a good example. But this is not only a competition based on quality itself; it includes marketing and sales activities as well as after-sales provision of warranty and maintenance service. There is a direct correlation between the satisfaction a consumer gets from vehicle servicing and the probability that the customer will be a repeat customer. In order to improve customer satisfaction, instill customer loyalty, and increase the dissemination of positive word-of-mouth by satisfied customers, a broad variety of things needs to be looked at.

Researchers N. P. Archer and G. O. Wesolowsky, both of the McMaster University of Hamilton, Ontario (1996), initially surveyed 5,000 motor vehicle owners. To measure customer satisfaction, independent agencies employed by motor vehicle manufacturers gathered data from owners on a regular basis. Owners were asked to list any critical positive or negative incidents they had experienced that related to the quality of their vehicle or to dealer service, or manufacturer policy on warranty support. The questions on these surveys concentrated not just on the vehicle itself, but also on a wide range of attributes including sales and service performance of dealers. It is stated that manufacturers attempt to improve customer loyalty to their vehicles yet dealer service is the weak link in car marketing.

The researchers took surveys of car owners of all makes of cars. The surveys asked questions on critical incidents involving product and service quality. These critical incidents are times when something happened involving either dealers or the vehicle itself, that stand out in the owners' minds. There was also information gathered about future intentions on automobile purchasing. In addition, owners were asked if they would recommend this manufacturer or this dealer to someone else.

The definition of quality in the eyes of manufacturers of durable goods is roughly a synonym for reliability and durability. The researchers found this definition to be defective since it fails to address customer perceptions of quality, which may differ from those of manufacturers. Objective quality must be differentiated from "perceived quality," which represents the consumer's judgement of the superiority of the product. These definitions refer to a high level of abstraction which may include several attributes. These attributes may be either intrinsic (determined by the physical composition of the product and learned by actual usage or consumption) or extrinsic (product-related but not a part of the product itself). Some intrinsic factors that may be used to evaluate quality are performance, reliability, durability, and image. Extrinsic attributes include price, warranty, advertising, and brand name. It was found that factory workers, managers, sales personnel, and consumers differ widely about which attributes they believe are best used to describe product quality. It is the service aspect of this that this research is about.

A customer's expectations of service may depend on the level of service that could be received from a competitor, or what advertising had led the customer to believe, or what the customer had historically received from this particular service. The interest in this study is the manner in which warranty service is performed. How this service is performed can affect the owner's perception of the dealer, the product and hence the manufacturer, with a potential impact on repeat sales. Survey responses of incidents called neutral, which accounted for 15 percent of responses, were eliminated since they don't contribute to opinion building. The rest of the survey responses were categorized into Significant or Not Significant choices. The survey pinpointed specific instances that owners may have faced.

The researchers found that owners tend to have a tolerance towards single negative vehicle incidents with regard to vehicle or manufacturer loyalty, but are not tolerant towards more than one such incident. However, negative service incidents can harm owner perceptions of both the dealer and the manufacturer. They found that more than one negative quality incident led to negative impacts on future intentions to acquire a similar vehicle or to acquire a vehicle from this manufacturer. A surprising find was that this does not carry over to the service aspect of ownership. A single negative service incident demonstrated a noticeably lower likelihood of owners to be loyal to vehicle or manufacturer. That implies that owners are relatively tolerant to vehicle glitches, but they lose patience if a dealer service is poor. Thus, positive vehicle incidents can help repair the damage to customer perceptions of negative vehicle incidents, but it takes a very good vehicle or manufacturer to counteract perceptions caused by poor dealer service. It was also found that there was a way of reversing negative incidents. The dealer is in a key position to proactively create service incidents and to avoid negative service incidents, thus improving customer loyalty to the dealer and counteracting negative vehicle incidents that affect loyalty to the manufacturer.

The implications of this study are important to any service organization as well as any firm expecting to do business in the coming years. Consumers have adapted to expect more for their money, and manufacturers do this by providing a sound product, along with the best available upkeep of the product. The method of evaluation that manufacturers use now is a start, but it doesn't break down problems into individual critical incidents. It is when problems are at this point, that it is easy for the manufacturer to quickly go about fixing the problem. Since critical incidents are likely to play a major role in the formation of customer opinion, it is essential that they be monitored and controlled as well as possible in order to improve the design quality of future products, thus maintaining a high level of confidence in the service provider's performance, and as a result, to increase the likelihood of repeat business. Makers of durable goods like computer hardware and software companies; industrial equipment and electronic equipment makers can use this information. The service aspect of business has always been a somewhat overlooked portion of doing business. It has always been important to sell items, with little attention paid to the quality of the service and the customer's satisfaction with the service. In today's competitive environment it is the sale of items, the satisfaction the consumer gets out of the product, and the service during the life of the product that is important.

6.4   RELATIONSHIPS, INVOLVEMENT, AND CUSTOMER SATISFACTION

Organizations must make adjustments based on interactions with their environment, as well as on internal actions, in order to survive. Therefore, how an organization interacts with its environment is critical. Customers are one group in an organization's environment. Organizations need to make sure that relationships with customers do not jeopardize the firm's survival. Measurements of customer satisfaction can be an indicator of an organization's relationship with its customers.

Professors Paul S. Goodman, Mark Fichman, and F. Javier Lerch at the Graduate School of Industrial Administration, Carnegie Mellon University, along with researcher Pamela R. Snyder (1995) studied the effects of core and peripheral aspects of customer-supplier relationships and customer involvement on overall customer satisfaction at the U.S. Postal Service (USPS). Participants in the analysis included 66 companies, in a metropolitan area in the Northeast each with at least $100,000 of annual business with the USPS.

Two hypotheses were tested in this study. The first, a two-part hypothesis, states that core factors (e.g., the product or service) and peripheral factors (e.g., firm responsiveness to inquiries) have a direct relationship with overall satisfaction. The first hypothesis also states that peripheral factors can affect satisfaction with core factors and in turn affect overall customer satisfaction. A questionnaire was used to investigate this hypothesis. Respondents were asked to rate their satisfaction with first class mail (core factor), as well as their satisfaction with account administration, account representative, inquiry handling (peripheral factors), overall customer satisfaction and intention to leave. The second hypothesis states that if customers who are dissatisfied with core factors and are highly involved with the firm, their overall dissatisfaction will be greater than customers who are less involved. The questionnaire looked at customer involvement in seven areas of the USPS' activities.

The results show several things. First, satisfaction with core factors has the strongest direct relationship with overall satisfaction. Peripheral factors are shown to be associated with overall satisfaction as well. Secondly, the model used by the researchers showed evidence that the satisfaction with the peripheral factors had an affect on the core factors and, in turn, on overall satisfaction. Finally, the researchers found that "respondents who are dissatisfied with first class mail and exhibit greater involvement in the relationship express greater overall dissatisfaction than those who are dissatisfied but less involved." In addition to this analysis, the researchers looked at the relationship between customer satisfaction and intention to leave. They found that dissatisfied respondents were more prone to switch under various cost savings scenarios than satisfied respondents.

Firms should look at their relationships with customers to determine likely affects of firm performance on customer satisfaction and retention. Depending on the situation, peripheral factors may be more critical and thus have a greater impact on core factors and overall satisfaction. Firms therefore should place equal emphasis on both types of factors when dealing with customers. Relationships with customers, and increasing customer involvement may have an impact on overall satisfaction as well. Managers should be cognizant of this information in decision making to improve changes for firm survival.

6.5 PAY LEVELS AND PRODUCT QUALITY

A small pay differential between lower-level employees (e.g. hourly workers and lower-level managers and professionals) may lead to high business-unit product quality, according to Professor Douglas Cowherd of the University of Michigan and Professor David Levine of the University of California, Berkeley (1992). On the other hand, a perception of injustice resulting from large pay differentials by lower-level workers can lead to a lessening of input and product quality.

The key result of the research was: product quality may be diminished when high salaries for the top managers are not matched by high wages for lower-level employees. Lower-level employees prefer smaller pay differentials than do upper-level managers. They compare their pay to that of higher-level groups and this comparison can result in feelings of equity (perceptions of being fairly treated) or inequity (those of unfair treatment). The degree of pay equity experienced by lower-employees can have a substantial influence on product quality by decreasing their commitment to top-management goals, effort, and cooperation. Individuals who believe they are treated fairly will have a stronger identification with their firm and thus commit to the company goals promoted by the top managers.

However, because the wage spread in North America and Western Europe is much larger than in Japan, lower-level workers still believe it is unjust if they factor in the upper levels' relatively high inputs (e.g., work efforts and skills). Also, product quality is a particularly important aspect of organizational effectiveness. Hence, it is critical to the economic performance of businesses to consider customer satisfaction. An organization's product quality is determined not just by managerial control systems based on record keeping, supervision, and inspection but also by lower-level employees' motivation, a factor that management cannot require or control. In this study, product quality is defined as customer perceptions of all non-price attributes of a company's goods and services (e.g., features, durability, delivery time, and after-sale service). Standard managerial control systems have greater influence on production quantity than on product quality because it is easier to monitor production by counting product units or through cost accounting than by assessing the many subtle factors of quality.

The researchers argue that lower-level employees are influenced by what they perceive as a more equitable distribution of rewards between themselves and higher level managers. Pay equity can substantially affect a worker's input because input is something within the worker's control. If they experience inequity, they are more likely to decrease their input, something over which they have control, rather than increase their output. Further, a perception of injustice creates resentment which can lead to less support for managerial goals and can even promote intense competition for promotions among lower-level workers. If this happens, product quality can suffer.

The researchers explored data on more than 500,000 employees in 102 business units in 41 corporations with headquarters in North America and Europe, primarily in the United States and Great Britain. Seventy-nine percent of the business units are primarily manufacturers. They operated in a variety of industries, such as stationery, cough drops, kitchen appliances, specialty inks, truck axles, boiler maintenance, and office equipment sales and service. Companies ranged in size from 59 to 90,000 employees. Data were supplied by general managers and the managers of finance, strategic planning, marketing, and human resources. This type of data sample and the statistical testing which the authors did clearly validate their findings.

What is also intriguing about this study is the number of issues which remain to be studied: (1) a comparison of the wages of lower-level workers with their co-workers, direct supervisors and similar/dissimilar groups; (2) the influence of other factors on product quality such as the political views of workers and the locus of control. Such studies would be helpful to the present one because it too is based on the perspective that organizational behavior is affected by both economic and social factors.

6.6 ASSESSING THE IMPACT OF TOTAL QUALITY MANAGEMENT EFFORTS

Hospitals and healthcare facilities in recent years have been under increased pressure to reduce costs and increase quality of care. In an effort to improve both of these factors, healthcare organizations are looking to utilize continuous quality improvement or total quality management. Improved efficiency and quality is achieved through continuous improvement, customer focus, structured processes, and organization wide-involvement. Does implementation of quality initiatives affect efficiency measures of hospitals and thereby affect the bottom line?

The following researchers were involved in this study: Stephen M. Shortell, James L. O'Brien, James M. Carman, and Richard W. Foster, Edward F. X. Hughes, Heidi Boerstler, and Edward J. O'Connor (1995). Their research evaluated hypothesis that included the positive benefits of continuous quality improvement/total quality management (CQI/TQM) implementation on human resources, patient outcomes, financial outcomes, and efficiency. The study sample included 61 hospitals affiliated with Western New York's Center for Health Management research. The average number of beds for each facility was 223 (181 national average). The hospitals were not selected randomly but are similar in size and occupancy to national averages.

The CEO and the person responsible for quality assurance within the respective hospital completed a questionnaire to determine whether the hospitals were using CQI/TQM. The following five criteria were used to assess this:

- Emphasis on processes instead of individuals
- Data-driven problem-solving approaches
- Use of cross-functional teams
- Customer focus

The results of this questionnaire indicated that 37 hospitals characterized themselves as users of CQI/TQM, while 24 indicated they utilized more traditional quality improvement efforts.

A 20-item questionnaire was used to measure organizational culture. The survey which was completed by up to 200 hospital employees, required respondents to distribute points among descriptions of what constitutes a group culture.

The approach that the hospitals used to implement quality improvement was measured by having the hospital's senior executives and quality assurance personnel respond to questions concerning the hospital is:

- Approach to change
- Administrative orientation
- Employee involvement
- Department involvement
- Physician involvement

The level of quality improvement implementation was measured using a questionnaire based on Malcolm Baldrige Criteria. The questions focused on leadership, information and analysis, human resource management, quality management, and strategic quality planning.

The first performance measure was an assessment by CEOs and Quality Directors of quality improvement impact on human resource development, patient outcomes, and financial results. The second measure was obtained through independently collected data concerning the length of stay and the charges for services of selected patient problems (i.e. pneumonia, stroke).

The results of this study indicated that the hospital culture and implementation approach is positively associated with a greater degree of quality improvement implementation. This means that hospitals that have cultures that can handle change, use teamwork philosophies, and have empowered employees are more likely to receive a higher degree of benefit from quality improvement implementation. Neither the size of the hospital (measured in number of beds) nor whether hospitals met all five of the criteria for being a CQI/TQM facility were significant in affecting implementation. The data further explains that a majority of the variation in the hospital's degree of implementation is attributed to the culture and implementation approach.

The studies of the performance measures show that quality improvement implementation has a significant effect on human resource development and patient outcomes but not on financial results. The analysis of the length of stay and charge measures revealed that larger hospitals have a higher length of stay and charge, while hospitals that were involved in all five criteria for a CQI/TQM site had a shorter length of stay and lower charge. It was also determined that larger hospitals were less likely to have a culture that is not suited to support implementation of quality improvement work.

The results indicated that there was not a direct correlation between quality improvement and financial results. It should be noted that this may be perceived in the short term since benefits can be intangible but when there is an improvement in human resource development and an increase in customer satisfaction, there will be positive financial benefits.

This study also indicates that the implementation of quality improvement initiatives in a large hospital is a difficult task. Before doing this in a large hospital, senior management needs to be aware of the issues and must take appropriate planning and implementation measures to ensure that the existing structure is addressed along with training of personnel to help foster change. Even though this has been proven to be a difficult task this study shows that there are incentives to undertake such an implementation. It appears that increasing customer satisfaction is the most significant effect, which is important for hospitals in the competitive environment that they face today. There are also implications from the results of this study for hospitals when considering long term strategic planning. There is significant support for hospitals to remain smaller in size in order to prevent a highly centralized structure. Senior management could look to ensure facilities remain small by specializing in certain technologies at certain sites along with a decentralized structure to help maintain a culture that is conducive to quality improvement efforts.

6.7 MANAGING THE QUALITY EFFORT IN A HOSPITAL SETTING

Americans will spend about 15 percent of the nation's gross domestic product on health care, the highest amount per capita among industrialized countries. However, the American public discontent with the poor quality of health care has been well documented. Approximately 40 percent of U.S. hospitals have attempted to adopt a quality improvement program. Successful implementation of such programs has been the exception rather than the rule.

The research described in the winter 1999 issue of *Health Care Management Review* presents a framework by which to effectively deploy a quality and customer orientation. M. M. Yasin, A. J. Czuchry, D. L. Jennings, and C. York, all of East Tennessee State University (1999), offer the efficient rapid assessment methodology (RAM) as a first step toward a complete total quality management (TQM) orientation in a health care setting.

RAM is proposed as a strategically driven assessment methodology designed to facilitate the initiation and expansion of the TQM process: RAM is based on the Malcolm Baldrige National Quality Award Criteria. The method can be conducted in a few hours for each category with relatively low cost, and recommendations generated from RAM can be immediately deployed. Although not as extensive as the TQM assessment methodology, RAM enables the collection of an extensive knowledge base. In order to facilitate the identification of key success factors and areas of opportunities for improvement, there must be a thorough understanding of the organizations' current operating and strategic realities. RAM gathers input from a focus group of internal and external entities, and then the input is categorized into strengths and opportunities for improvement (OFI). The OFI are then prioritized into workable action plans for deployment. Internal and external benchmarks guide the implementation and monitoring of the action plans. The results of RAM can be used to provide the documentation required for a complete TQM orientation.

The research team was approached by the administrative team of a mid-sized, private, not-for-profit, tertiary hospital for assistance in examining the hospital's TQM effort to date. It, like many other hospitals, had not realized many of the operational and strategic benefits hoped for with their TQM implementation. The hospital is regional, licensed for 407 inpatient beds, has nearly 100,000 annual inpatient days and more than 115,000 annual outpatient visits.

A preliminary analysis revealed four primary opportunities for improvement:

1. goals needed to be more strategically aligned;
2. the public needed to be more aware of the hospital's quality efforts;
3. a more systematic approach to the quality effort was needed to ensure synergy and avoid suboptimization; and
4. more integration and coordination was needed in the TQM effort and processes.

After the preliminary analysis, the researchers used RAM to conduct a rapid assessment of the hospital's quality approach. A leadership focus group was conducted in July 1995. Leadership-oriented questions developed by the Juran Institute were given to for the focus group, eliciting responses which were then categorized into focused areas such as customer focus and financial efficiency.

Focus group participants discovered that each group had their own unique definition of quality and that these definitions should be synthesized. The common theme among OFI concerned the need for improved communication. Enhanced vertical and horizontal communication and the linking of TQM communication with strategy were specific areas cited for improvement. Also, the need for an evaluation of TQM communication effectiveness and efficiency was noted.

RAM is a practical process that allows health care organizations to become quality oriented without the full investment required for a TQM strategy. RAM provides organizations a way to begin systematic thinking about quality, while simultaneously facilitating the initial step toward a TQM orientation.

6.8   CAN TQM REALLY IMPROVE THE BOTTOM LINE?

After years of emphasis on total quality management (TQM) programs, it has been left primarily to speculation as to whether or not they provide financial benefits to a firm upon implementation. Will improved quality lead to better sales and greater profits, or simply be another expense? The answer, according to some recent research, appears to be a mixture of both.

Kevin Hendricks of The College of William and Mary, and Vinod Singhal of the Georgia Institute of Technology (1997) have compared the financial operating performances of companies winning quality awards against other companies of similar size and industry. They tested the general hypothesis that implementing effective TQM programs improves the operating performance of firms. By looking at the data before and after the years of the award for these companies, they hoped to develop empirical evidence of the financial impact of TQM programs.

The study consisted of an evaluation of publicly available financial accounting data over a ten year period for nearly 400 publicly traded firms that won their first quality award between 1983 and 1993. The winning of quality awards was viewed as a measure of validity that the firms had effectively implemented TQM programs. (By using the assessment of an independent third party, they avoided the biases associated with asking the firms to judge themselves and their results.) Control samples were also identified based on size, industry, and availability of the required financial data. By using the data for the control group as a comparison, the researchers were able to benchmark financial performance and account for any potential economic or industry-wide influences.

Using three general concepts of TQM as a basis, hypotheses about expected fiscal performance were developed for each one. The first, cost of quality, suggests that fewer defectives will increase profits (through reduced losses of goods). This generated the hypothesis that implementing an effective TQM program will improve the profitability of the firm. The primary financial measure used for this was operating income before depreciation. The second, total customer satisfaction, suggests that customers will be willing to pay more or buy more, and therefore revenues will increase. Net sales was the primary financial measure used to test the second hypothesis, that implementing an effective TQM program will increase revenues. The third, organizational innovation, suggests that human and physical assets will be utilized more productively, thereby reducing costs. The third hypothesis then was that implementing an effective TQM program will reduce costs, measured primarily by cost per dollar of sales. Other measures were also looked at, including capital expenditure, total assets, and number of employees, that were not linked to any specific hypotheses.

Results tend to indicate that overall financial performance improves with the implementation of TQM programs, compared to the results of the control group. There is strong evidence that firms having won quality awards outperform the control sample on operating income-based measures.

From six years before until three years after winning the award, the mean change in operating income was 107% higher than that of the control sample. In addition, reasonably strong evidence exists showing that such firms outperform the control sample in sales growth. During the same time period of six years before until three years after winning an award, revenues were almost 64% higher. Finally, there is weak evidence showing that test sample firms are more successful at reducing costs. The mean change in cost per dollar of sales was 1.27 percentage points lower over the ten year time period than for the control group. It was also found that the test sample firms did increase their rates of capital expenditures and experienced higher growth in employment and total assets than those in the control group.

These results are significant for many firms considering whether or not to implement a TQM program. Evidence has now supported the hypothesis that implementing an effective TQM program will improve the operating performance of a firm. While the costs of implementation can be very real and often high, these programs provide benefits which easily outweigh their costs. The concern of some business managers that the direct and indirect costs of implementing such programs are too high is simply not founded. TQM should not be viewed as just another fad, but rather as an effective tool for not only improving quality but also for enhancing the financial performance of a firm. This will make both customers and shareholders happy.

REFERENCES

Archer, N. P., & Wesolowsky, G. O. (1996). Consumer response to service and product quality: A study of motor vehicle owners. *Journal of Operations Management, 14*(2), 103-118.

Cowherd D. M., & Levine, D. I. (1992). Product quality and pay equity between lower-level employees and top management: An investigation of distributive justice theory. *Administrative Science Quarterly, 37*(2), 302-320.

Goodman, P. S., Fichman, M., Lerch, F. J., & Snyder, P. R. (1995). Customer-firm relationships, involvement, and customer satisfaction. *Academy of Management Journal, 38*(5), 1310-1315.

Harvey, J. (1998). Service quality: A tutorial. *Journal of Operations Management, 16,* 583-597.

Hendricks K. B., & Singhal, V. R. (1997), Does implementing an effective TQM program actually improve operating performance? Empirical evidence from firms that have won quality awards. *Management Science, 43*(9), 1258-1274.

Shortell, S. M., O'Brien, J. L., Carman, J. M., Foster, R. W., Hughes, E. F. X., Boerstler, H., & O'Connor, E. J. (1995). Assessing the impact of continuous quality improvement/total quality management: Concept versus implementation. *Health Services Research, 30*(2), 377-401.

Weiner, B. J., Shortell, S. M., & Alexander, J. (1997). Promoting clinical involvement in hospital quality improvement efforts: The effects of top management, board, and physician leadership. *Health Services Research, 32*(4), 491-510.

Yasin, M. M., Czuchry, A. C., Jennings, D. L., & York, C. (1999). Managing the quality effort in a health care setting: An application. *Health Care Management Review, 24*(1), 45-56.

CHAPTER 7

CONTINUOUS QUALITY IMPROVEMENT IN HEALTH SYSTEMS

This chapter addresses continuous improvement in general and in a few cases specifically in health care. It is essentially a continuation of the previous chapter on total quality management.

The first study describes a study to validate the Malcolm Baldrige National Quality Award (MBNQA) criteria to evaluate improvement and overall quality efforts in a firm. Tens of thousands of firms annually use these criteria to evaluate those managerial, quality, technical, operating, and leadership qualities that determine how well the firm is doing in term of overall quality and operating performance. Since there is no data available on the validity of the NBNQA criteria they used the Arizona Governor's Quality Award (AGQA) criteria for which data were available. Through statistical testing they found that the two sets of quality criteria were very similar, and the AGQA data could therefore be used to validate the MBNQA criteria. Their conclusion was that managers who follow continuous quality improvement management approaches as outlined by the MBNQA model criteria are likely to produce good operational results and customer satisfaction.

Proven Solutions for Improving Health and Lowering Health Care Costs, pages 97–109.
Copyright © 2003 by Information Age Publishing, Inc.
All rights of reproduction in any form reserved.
ISBN: 1-59311-000-6 (paper), 1-59311-001-4 (cloth)

The second study is an impact study of the use of both technological utilization and employee participation and empowerment on economic performance of the firm. The study was based on a survey of 268 manufacturing firms. The researcher found that individually high technological utilization had a significant positive impact on company performance. Also employee participation and empowerment by itself had a significant positive impact on company performance. But the maximum benefit in terms of economic performance was achieved by those firms that combined high technological utilization and extensive employee participation and empowerment.

The third study is a comparative audit of surgical practices by surgeons in hospitals in the North West Thames region of the United Kingdom. The focus of the study was on appendectomies. The 19 clinicians studied were responsible for 10,214 hospital discharges or deaths, including 415 cases where appendectomy was the primary procedure. The two inputs studied consisted of patient age and sex. The three outputs studied consisted of length of hospital stay, use of prophylactic antibiotics and proportion of patients with an abnormal appendix removed. The results showed that mean length of stay was 4.6 days with a range from 2.1 to 7.6 days. Several surgeons had average length of stay considerably longer than the mean. The overall rate of prophylactic antibiotic use was 38 percent with one surgeon treating 85 percent of his cases. Abnormal appendices removed were reported as 67%, meaning one third of appendectomies were unnecessary. The study indicates that considerable savings could be realized if better diagnostic technology was available, and if surgeons stayed closer to the norm in terms of hospital length of stay and prophylactic antibiotic use.

The fourth study asked if a total quality management program improves quality performance. Prior research has identified eight critical factors of quality management. They were:

1. role of management leadership and policy;
2. role of the quality department;
3. employee training;
4. product or service design;
5. supplier quality management;
6. process management;
7. quality data and reporting; and
8. employee relations.

A survey asking input on the eight factors was sent to about 300 aerospace firms with an 84 percent response rate. The results indicate that a company should not assume that simply installing a quality improvement process will by itself improve quality performance. It is important that implementation of the process by all affected parties as opposed to just installation is the critical success factor.

The fifth study focuses on the quality of community nursing services in the United Kingdom. The objective of the study was to measure the quality of nursing services as perceived by the consumer. Data for the study was collected from three sources: customer interviews, questionnaires, and observations in field notes. Three types of nurses were evaluated: district nurses, health visitors, and school nurses. Three categories of quality measurement formed the focus consisting of technical, interface, and environment. The results of the study indicated that the district nurses ranked their main roles as looking after people who are sick and visiting them in their homes. The health visitors' roles were mainly seen as checking and advising on the normal development and progress of infants. The school nurses' roles were viewed differently by the mothers, the teachers, and the students. Mothers wanted the nurses' assessment of the normal progress and development of their children. Teachers viewed the nurses' roles as doing preventive work and important in health education. The students viewed the nurses' roles as checking normal progress, immunization, and health education. The study is important in its goal to discover what each recipient of the service perceives as being important.

The sixth study addresses quality's impact on learning as measured by the classical learning curve first used in the aircraft industry during the 1930s. The learning curve projects time to do a task or cost to perform a task. Task cost or time declines by a fixed percentage each time output is doubled. Over the years the main milestone of the learning curve has been cumulative output, and it has been tested out and found useful in many applications. In this case the authors propose to apply the curve, not to cumulative output, but to the reduction in defectives produced or errors made. The results show that the reduction of defectives produced or errors made produces a steeper curve than the curve based on the classical cumulative output measurement.

In this chapter we have covered six quality-related studies which are either in health care or have clear implications for work in the health care field. All studies show, when implemented properly, continuous quality improvement efforts produce results.

7.1 THE VALIDATION OF THE MALCOLM BALDRIGE NATIONAL QUALITY AWARD AND ITS IMPACT ON BUSINESS

Tens of thousand of firms have used the Malcolm Baldrige National Quality Award (MBNQA) criteria to improve the quality of their products and processes since its conception in 1988. The MBNQA was a godsend to managers who had long been in need of a model to define the extent of effort necessary for complete organizational quality and a means for evaluating progress toward becoming a world-class competitor in quality products and services. But the MBNQA has never been validated. Is the MBNQA a valid model that the manager can adopt with confidence that the criteria are appropriate measures for a total quality improvement strategy? From 1988 to 1995, over a million copies of the MBNQA criteria have been requested from the National Institute of Standards and Technology. With such a vast number of organizations using these unvalidated criteria to assess their own organizational quality, this research addresses an important question.

The ultimate objective of this research is to provide evidence of the validity of the MNBQA criteria. Research was conducted by Gertrude P. Pannirselvam, School of Business, Southern Illinois University at Edwardsville, Sue P. Siferd and William A. Ruch, both of the College of Business, Arizona State University (1998).

Since the data from the MNBQA award process are confidential, an alternate source for suitable data had to be found. Many states have developed quality award programs patterned on the MBNQA criteria. The Arizona Governor's Quality Award (AGQA) was found to be sufficiently close to the MBNQA in all respects. In fact, one of the researchers was involved in the early formation of the Baldrige Award and served as a Baldrige examiner for several years and also spearheaded the design effort for the AGQA. The evaluation process used for the AGQA is as similar as possible to the process used for the MBNQA.

The researchers compared the MBNQA criteria to two other instruments that measure quality management practices. The two other instruments are the Saraph, et al. model and the Flynn, et al. model. The Saraph, et al. instrument was based on the concepts of quality gurus such as Deming, Juran, and Crosby. The Flynn, et al instrument is based on the practitioner literature in quality management. While all three models have many items in common, each of the instruments has a different target and objective for evaluation. The MBNQA criteria are found to be more comprehensive and less prescriptive than the other instruments. In the MBNQA model there is a greater emphasis on continuous improvement, customer focus, and strategic quality planning. However, the other instruments are validated and the MBNQA is not.

The researchers next examined content validity, construct validity and predictive validity. Content validity for MBNQA criteria was established by comparing several leading quality management philosophies to MBNQA categories. Construct and predictive validity were tested using data from AGQA. The results indicate that the items in each category belong together and, hence, have construct validity. Predictive validity was tested by performing a correlation between items in the approach set and items in the results set. The high correlation found between the two sets indicated predictive validity.

The AGQA model is a reliable and valid measure of organizational quality. Because the AGQA so closely resembles the MBNQA, the generalization may be made that the MBNQA model may be used with confidence by researchers studying organizational quality.

The implications of this study for business are twofold. The MBNQA serves as a template for creating organizational quality. It also provides a way to measure and evaluate the quality efforts of the organization. The validity analysis shows that all items in each category play a role in achieving excellence. If a manager were to concentrate on only one or two of these quality improvement areas, his efforts would be less than effective. Managers who follow total quality management approaches as outlined by the MBNQA model criteria are likely to produce good operational results and customer satisfaction.

While the MBNQA model and criteria may never be validated directly, it does have a scientific foundation and may be used with confidence.

7.2 MANUFACTURING TECHNOLOGY, EMPLOYEE PARTICIPATION, AND ECONOMIC PERFORMANCE

This paper focuses on the relationship between manufacturing technology and employee-related programs. Traditionally these two functions have been viewed as completely separate entities. Technology-driven strategies are viewed as an improvement of economic performance by decreasing labor costs and increasing managerial control. Investments in employee participation programs, on the other hand, are often viewed with skepticism and are seen as increasing costs and diffusing control. The purpose of the study in this article is to show the benefit of the improvement of technology while simultaneously increasing employee participation.

The study was conducted by researcher George Gyan-Baffour (1994), who surveyed 268 managers in a mid-western State. The managers represented many industries including primary metals, metal fabrication, industrial machinery, electronics, transportation equipment, and engineering instrumentation. Of the 268 surveys completed, 60 percent were completed by plant managers, 16 percent were completed by industrial relations or human resource managers, and 24 percent were completed by various other managers.

The author of the study was trying to determine the economic impact of a company which increases its investment in technology, increases employee participation programs, and implements both technology and employee participation programs simultaneously.

The amount of technology a company utilizes was determined by the number of advanced machine tools used (such as numerical control and computerized numerical control). Employee participation was determined by answers to such questions as degree of worker involvement in production decisions, worker training programs, and the implementation of new technology.

The four worker participation measures used to determine the level of employee involvement were participation in strategic decision making, capacity to participate, technical skill formation, and productivity information acquisition. The performance measures used in the study included process quality, production flexibility, and productivity change. The research methodology consisted of a statistical analysis of the answers from the questionnaires along with derived scores from the worker participation measures.

The background theory for this study originated in many previous studies that show that technology in the workplace and employee programs benefit the company in various areas, but these two factors were never before researched together. It is the author's theory that companies are not maximizing the value of new technology if employee involvement is low.

The researcher gathered three major conclusions from his research. The first finding is that the level of advanced technology has a significant positive influence on all measured performance variables. This suggests that the companies with the highest technological level will have a competitive advantage with all else being equal.

The second finding shows that employee participation has a significant positive impact on both quality and production flexibility.

The third result is that the maximum benefit in all areas was found in firms that have both extensive manufacturing technology and extensive employee participation programs.

The implications of this paper are that it puts in focus the need to utilize the power of the work force to benefit the company. Utilizing advanced technology is no longer enough in today's global competitive marketplace. More emphasis is being placed on quality and production flexibility than ever before. Employee empowerment goes hand in hand with technology in meeting these competitive pressures.

7.3   COMPARATIVE AUDIT BETWEEN HOSPITALS: THE EXAMPLE OF APPENDECTOMY

The practice of medical and health care varies remarkably between countries, regions within countries, cities, hospitals, and individual practitioners. In this paper the authors describe a comparison of diagnoses and surgical practices by surgeons in the North West Thames region of England. The focus of the study is on appendectomies.

Researchers N. A. Black and L. Moore of the Health Services Research Unit, Department of Public Health and Policy, London School of Hygiene and Tropical Medicine in London (1994) used data collected through a comparative audit system they developed during the late 1980s in the North West Thames region of the U.K.

The data collected from 14 general surgeons and five urologists working in nine National Health Service Hospitals in the North West Thames region during the January to June 1990 period.

During the collection period the clinicians were responsible for 10,214 discharges or deaths, including 415 cases in which appendectomy was the primary procedure. Two surgeons with fewer than 10 appendectomies were eliminated from the sample leaving 17 surgeons with an average of 23.6 appendectomy cases per surgeon for a total sample size of 401.

The two inputs studied consisted of patients' ages and sex ratio. The three outputs studied consisted of length of hospital stay, use of prophylactic antibiotics, and proportion of appendectomy patients having an abnormal appendix removed.

The results of the input variable analysis showed that the average age of the patient was 25 years with little variation between the average patient ages by surgeon, except for a low outlier (average of 19) and a high outlier (average age of 36). Women consisted of 54 percent of the sample with considerable variations among the surgeons, ranging from 30 percent to 75 percent.

The output variables showed considerably more variation, and this raises clinical practice questions. The overall mean length of stay was 4.6 days, ranging from 2.1 to 7.6 days per patient, with several surgeons having average length of stays considerably longer than the overall mean. Use of prophylactic antibiotics showed considerable variation with two surgeons reporting no use and one surgeon treating 85 percent of his cases. The overall rate of prophylactic antibiotic use was 38 percent. Abnormal appendices removed were reported as 67 percent, indicating that one third of appendectomies were unnecessary, at least at that point in time. One surgeon reported 40 percent of abnormal appendices, increasing the mean proportion of the other surgeons to 80 percent, a more excessive figure. Only four surgeons reported wound infections occurring in 2 to 4 percent of patients, thus raising the issue of prophylactic use of antibiotics.

The results of this study indicate that an institutionalized form of medical and surgical procedure reporting can reveal considerably useful information in terms of quality of care. Retrospectively, surgeons not conforming to norms of their peers can be made aware of their practices and if appropriate admonished to improve their practices. Prospectively, standards can be established for surgeons, based on accepted practices in their profession as practiced by their peers. In terms of diagnosis, the study indicates that considerable savings could be realized if improved diagnostic procedures and technology were available.

7.4 DOES A TOTAL QUALITY MANAGEMENT PROGRAM IMPROVE QUALITY PERFORMANCE?

The relationships between a company and their suppliers are crucial in today's business environment. Operational strategies such as just in time production, inventory management, and production management require close cooperation between manufacturer and supplier. Similarly, it is crucial for a company focused on building a quality product that the parts supplied to them by supplier companies are of the same high quality. Otherwise, the costs involved in rework and order delays become excessive. L. B. Forker's research at the Boston University School of Management (1997) set out to test three hypothesis that focus on the quality of product supplied to the aerospace industry. The three hypotheses were:

1. Total quality management (TQM) implementation in intermediate manufacturing facilities is positively related to quality performance.
2. The interaction of process optimization (efficiency) and extent of TQM implementation is positively related to quality performance.
3. Bilateral dependence, a reflection of transaction specific investments made by the buyer and supplier firms, will be negatively related to quality performance.

There had been numerous other research studies prior to this paper and they had collectively recognized eight critical factors of quality management:

1. Role of management leadership and quality policy,
2. Role of the quality department,
3. Training,
4. Product and Service design,
5. Supplier quality management,
6. Process management,
7. Quality data and reporting, and
8. Employee relations.

These factors were utilized in this present study to test the hypotheses. Two hundred and ninety aerospace firms were identified and surveyed on questions relating to the above factors with an 84 percent response rate.

The statistical results showed mixed support for the hypotheses. First, there was no direct support that the extent of TQM implementation solely at a supplier site increased the quality performance of their product. Secondly, TQM implementation in conjunction with high levels of process optimization, particularly the role of top management and supplier efficiency, strongly coincided with the level of quality performance. Thirdly, the level of customer and/or supplier dependence did not affect the quality of product supplied. The suppliers felt that quality was not a major determinant by their largest customers in placing orders with them in comparison to the price that they could offer. This belief was widespread throughout the aerospace industry.

The data collected also shows a strong correlation between the amount of training that is provided to associates and the increased performance in the area of quality. This is not overly surprising and is assumed to be true in this industry. The main focus of this paper reflects that a company should not assume that simply installing a TQM process in their plants will alone improve their quality performance. It is also necessary to implement a TQM process with process optimization to increase efficiencies. These two combined approaches provide a quality environment and enhanced tools and processes to improve overall quality and efficiency.

7.5 QUALITY OF COMMUNITY NURSING SERVICES IN UNITED KINGDOM

Community Health, which is one of the health authorities in the United Kingdom (UK), was contacted for a project to measure the quality of nursing services as perceived by the consumer. The reason for this study was to clarify a debate that was taking place in the UK on the quality of nursing services. A consultant, Lucy Gaster, was contracted to help prepare a literature search for the project by gathering all of the data from different groups of people on the quality areas of technical, interface, and environmental aspects of nursing services in an aritcle by Gott and Peckham (1993).

Gaster grouped the study in various categories: district nurses, health visitors, and school nurses. Data was collected from three sources: customer interviews, questionnaires, and observation field notes. The overall goal was to see how the consumers of these different groups viewed the quality of the health care from these nurses. This would help the UK determine what areas will need improvement in the area of nursing for the health care industry. In the area of district nursing, 4 customers were interviewed; 16 out of 30 questionnaires were collected; and 3 district nurses' treatment sessions were observed. For the health visitors, 12 mothers were interviewed; 18 out of 30 questionnaires were collected; and 3 clinics were observed. Finally, for the school nurses, 12 mothers, 12 teachers, and 3 secondary school classes were interviewed; 15 out of 30 questionnaires were collected; and 3 school nurses were observed.

Gaster had each of the areas (interviews, questionnaires, and field notes) focus on three categories of quality measurement: technical, interface, and environment. In addition, for the questionnaires and the interviews, people were free to respond to the ranking of the five roles that Gaster thought were important nursing roles. The roles are:

1. giving care to sick people,
2. screening and immunizing to prevent disease,
3. verifying that people are progressing/developing normally,
4. teaching people how to live a healthy lifestyle, and
5. influencing local businesses, councilors, shopkeepers, etc. for healthy public places.

Then, the rankings were compared to see how the different customer groups viewed the importance of nursing. This information helps the UK understand where the problems are in viewing the quality of nursing.

Studies indicated that the district nurses ranked their main roles as looking after people who are sick and visiting them in their rooms or homes. For the category of interface, these nurses generally see elderly people who cannot get to the doctor's office or people who have been recently released from the hospital. Interview evidence suggested that more of these nurses were needed. One of the candidates responded that this short staff problem is probably an issue with the "higher-ups." The technical aspect of their service was praised highly for efficiency, and effectiveness, and the service as being delivered by very knowledgeable people. The district nurse clinics were observed as being friendly and the nurses had good interpersonal skills. Finally, for the area of environment, there was a home-like feel to the clinics, and for agencies whose nurses go to homes clients enjoy the fact that they do not have to go to see the doctor weekly.

Studies conducted on the health visitors' roles were mainly seen as checking and advising on the normal development and progress of infants. In the area of interface, the health visitors were seen as mentors or as guides to give mothers advice on certain questions or procedures on new babies. Some people viewed these health visitors as policewomen or social workers and feared that they would have their children taken away from them. As for the technical aspect, the ease of contacting the health visitors (efficiency) was viewed as very good; however, the advice that was given by them was sometimes conflicting with the mothers' viewpoints. The environment of the clinics was reported as cheerful with adequate resources, but there was a concern by some mothers that there was no playroom for toddlers to keep them busy. The quality of the service at the clinics was also rated highly.

Finally, studies indicated that the viewpoint on the school nurses' roles were different among the mothers, teachers, and students. The mothers sought these nurses for assessing normal progress and development; while the teachers viewed the nurses' role as preventive work and important in health education. The students viewed the nurses' role as checking normal progress, immunizing, and health education. For the area of interface, parents stated that there is a community problem between the nurses and the parents. Some parents stated that problems are not addressed to the parents about their child. The teachers suggested that there is not enough information given to the nurses as to where they can obtain new information to help the children. The students stated that some felt fairly comfortable talking to the nurse and others were glad to have a nurse at their school to listen to their problems. The technical aspect of these nurses was ranked as efficient and they used effective procedures, but more information is needed for the parents on all of the services that a school can provide for their children. The environment at the clinic locations range from warm and friendly to adequate.

This study on the health care industry in the UK will help in assessing the quality of care that skilled nurses are providing to their customers. Total quality management practices are important to an industry so that certain procedures are applied to in the same way throughout their various organizations. For instance, communication seems to be a common problem among the health visitors and the school nurses, but the district nurses were viewed as very knowledgeable and communicative. Another area of quality determination is the area of efficiency and effectiveness. It was noted that care provided was acceptable in all areas, but customers noted that more nurses are needed to meet the daily demand. All of the findings help the health care industry assess what is important to their customers today and in the future, and what areas need improvement.

7.6 QUALITY'S IMPACT ON LEARNING

Quality of goods manufactured may be linked to learning. Research suggests that quality increases over time if defective units have greater impact than good units on learning and vice versa. It is useful to examine the empirical evidence found to answer questions that arise. These questions are:

1. Is cumulative output of the defective or good units statistically significant in explaining learning curve effects?
2. Do defective and good units help explain learning effects equally and if not, which one has greater explanatory power?
3. How can traditional learning curve models be modified to take into account the impact of quality levels on learning?

The experience gained over time, as a firm produces more units of a product, leads to reductions in the unit cost of production, owing to reductions in labor, machine hours and material costs. This phenomenon is referred to as a learning curve. Learning curves have several applications in areas such as pricing, anticipating competitive behavior, planning, forecasting, marketing and manufacturing strategy. Individual learning curves may differ across firms within the same industry. Little is known about why there is considerable variation in the rate at which different firms learn.

Studies of Japanese manufacturing firms suggest that quality-related managerial activities might be an important factor in explaining the differences in learning rates across firms. When defect levels are high, a firm needs to devote additional effort to investigate the cause of defects. This leads to additional knowledge of the manufacturing process, which results in increased quality and productivity. In this process, the defective output may be seen as a trigger for improvement efforts that result in increased learning effects. Thus, the study of Japanese manufacturing firms provides a basis for the theoretical argument that firms choosing to produce high quality products will learn faster, or go down a steeper learning curve, than firms producing lower quality products.

The relationship between quality and learning is best explained within the framework of induced and autonomous learning. Autonomous learning involves automatic improvements that result from sustained production, and reaping its limited benefits requires little conscious managerial effort. Traditional learning curve models operate under the assumption of autonomous learning, and use cumulative output as a proxy for production knowledge and experience. In contrast to autonomous learning, induced learning represents the result of deliberate actions taken by management, workers, and engineers to improve quality and efficiency in the production process. A quality based learning curve model would use cumulative defective output (rather than total cumulative output) as a proxy for production knowledge and experience. Quality concerns provoke induced learning, which is understood to achieve greater learning curve effects.

An empirical study was conducted to examine the impact of quality on learning. The focus of the study was on three questions: 1. How well does cumulative output of defective good units explain learning curve effects? 2. Do defective units explain learning curve effects better than good units? 3. How should cumulative experience be represented in the learning curve model when the quality level may have an impact on learning effects?

The researchers Li and Rajagopalan (1997) collected data from two firms, referred to as A and B. Firm A is labor intensive and produces tire treading, and Firm B is more labor intensive and produces a variety of medical instruments. They collected monthly data over a period of three years for Firm A and a period of two and a half years for Firm B. They measured defective rates along with direct labor hours worked and output for each of the firms.

They tested the three questions with empirical data collected and came to the following conclusions. They found that cumulative output of good units explain learning curve effects. Also found was that defective units help explain learning curve benefits. Their research also led them to conclude that defective units are more significant than good units in explaining learning curve effects. After testing their last hypothesis, they concluded that both Firm A and Firm B could change some production procedures to modify defective output and the curves associated with them.

The impact of defective and good units on learning can be explained as follows. If there is a period of defective products, managers will take notice and all efforts are concentrated on correcting the problem. These efforts lead to a better understanding and can help improve quality in the future. It can also lead to process changes, which will require less labor, and fewer other resources. After a product is manufactured for a while, defect levels decrease so learning will also slow down.

This study, in essence, can help managers decide whether or not processes need to be changed and also how learning from production of defective items can be more helpful than learning from good units. The increased knowledge can assist the manager in increasing productivity by reducing labor hours and other resources consumed in the production process.

REFERENCES

Black N. A., & Moore, L. (1994). Comparative audit between hospitals: The example of appendectomy. *International Journal of Health Care Quarterly Assurance,* 7(3), 11-15.

Forker, L. B. (1997). Factors affecting supplier quality performance. *Journal of Operations Management, 15,* 243-269.

Gott, M., & Packham, H. (1993). The quality of community nursing services: Report of an exploratory study in a UK health authority. *International Journal of Health Care Quarterly Assurance, 6*(1), 24-31.

Gyan-Baffour, G. (1994). Advanced manufacturing technology, employee participation and economic performance: An empirical analysis. *Journal of Managerial Issues, 15*(6), 491.

Li, G., & Rajagopalan, S. (1997). The impact of quality on learning. *Journal of Operations Management, 15*(3), 181-191.

Pannirselvam, G. P., Siferd, S. P., & Ruch, W. A. (1998). Validation of the Arizona governor's quality award criteria: A test of the Baldrige criteria. *Journal of Operations Management, 16,* 529-550.

CHAPTER 8

OPERATIONS MANAGEMENT IN HEALTH SERVICES

This chapter addresses the issues of services and operations including manpower scheduling, resource requirement planning, staffing levels, project management, transportation, supplies management, and purchasing.

The first study explores planning resource requirements in health care organizations. The focus of the study is on using queuing or waiting line analysis to help solve many resource requirements planning problems. Queuing can be very useful to determine capacity but also in planning the utilization of the available capacity in the health care setting. The benefit of the approach is that it allows management to determine the optimal tradeoff between available capacity and client waiting time in the health care system.

The second study also utilizes queuing or waiting line analysis to study how alternate level of care (ALC) patients can be most effectively placed following discharge from an acute care facility. ALC patients who are backed up in acute care facilities are responsible for elevating health care costs. The proposed model is able to assist policy makers to determine the optimal number of ALC beds required in a community.

The third study presents an evaluation model of outpatient appointment scheduling using simulation. The model used is also a queuing or

Proven Solutions for Improving Health and Lowering Health Care Costs, pages 111–125.
Copyright © 2003 by Information Age Publishing, Inc.
All rights of reproduction in any form reserved.
ISBN: 1-59311-000-6 (paper), 1-59311-001-4 (cloth)

waiting line problem but by using simulation a better approximation to reality is obtained. The researchers point out that people have low tolerance for long waiting times and improved patient scheduling rules need to be implemented in order to allow better client service while at the same time minimizing provider idle time.

The fourth study addresses the issue of nurse staffing levels in U.S. hospitals. The specific focus of this study was on the relationship between nurse staffing and nurse-sensitive events versus non-nurse sensitive events. Five nurse-sensitive events were identified and four non-nurse sensitive events. The research found significant inverse relationships between nurse staffing and post-operative nurse-sensitive events. Also large hospitals were found to have significantly lower specific nurse-sensitive events than small hospitals. The researchers conclude that staffing levels should be based on the volume of nurse-sensitive events that can be anticipated and not just on number of beds or on number of patients.

The fifth study focuses on high-performing project management organizations in the pharmaceutical industry. The study was designed to determine how various approaches to project management affect organizational performance and how to identify critical success factors for managing projects. The researchers found that project team variables such as priority for resources and team size were significantly related to performance. Larger teams with high priority for resources performed better than teams which did not have those benefits. Also emotional attachment to the project by team members and matrix-structured teams, in which the team members report both to their functional department and to the project leader, produced more effective performance.

The sixth study was also a team study. The team in this case was a manufacturing work team. The researchers found that teams with highly trained workers with high seniority, and high levels of cohesion performed better and had higher gains in both labor productivity and quality.

The seventh study explores the effectiveness of high performance work systems (HPWS) increasingly being used in organizations. HPWS are not well defined but all have the objective to improve effectiveness, efficiency, quality, and worker satisfaction. The researchers found that HPWS must be selected, developed, and implemented carefully. Secondly, they found that companies must adopt a HPWS that is capable of changing within the organization. Third, companies must be patient because it may take some time for benefits to emerge.

The eighth study reports on a study of purchasing practices and just-in-time (JIT) operations. The researchers found that JIT producers put greater emphasis on product performance and product quality. Also JIT users had a higher interaction rate than non-JIT users with inventory management, transportation providers, and engineering.

In this chapter we have summaries of eight papers in services and operations which have either specific references to health care or are direct studies of health care situations. The major question addressed in nearly every study was the degree of effectiveness that could be achieved.

8.1 PLANNING IN HEALTH CLINICS AND BLOOD BANKS

More emphasis is being placed on resource productivity and service provided to patients due to the changes in health care resources which are ever more limited and expensive. Operationally health care needs focus on capacity planning which means meeting goals of high service quality and high resource utilization. The real need is to take into consideration the probabilistic nature of health care systems while using optimization to quantify customer service levels. There are very few studies in the health care field using the techniques of queuing and optimization.

Researchers Bretthauer and Cote (1998) demonstrate how a basic model used in the health care system for planning resource requirements fits a health maintenance organization (HMO) clinic and a blood bank. A method is shown to demonstrate how to derive a sample solution. The example points out the tradeoff relationship between average patient waiting time and capacity costs. The capacity planning model also used an algorithm that solved the problem via computer. For expected changes in patient arrival rates, performance criteria, and resources, a multi-period extension was developed.

To illustrate the planning capacity model a blood bank and a HMO clinic are used as examples. A blood bank needs to know how many donation stations are required and the number of nursing and support staff needed. Capacity needs to be sufficient without lengthy waiting times for donors. Also, there needs to be a balance between high capacity and low costs. Similar decision levels for equipment, staff, and service levels are required for an HMO clinic. How many physicians should be on duty, how are nurse's aides allocated, and how are exam rooms utilized based on daily patient arrivals is the main concern for HMO clinic administrators.

An optimization/queuing network model was developed to determine resource requirements, so that capacity costs are kept to a minimum by using a set of performance constraints. The HMO clinic is based on real data collected from a large HMO. Service times and arrivals are configured using queuing stations to take into account the probabilistic nature that is typical in health care systems. The length of time to provide service to a patient and the realization that a patient may not show up for an appointment or may be late is what is meant by probabilistic nature. Service levels are measured by constraints utilizing optimization methods.

The capacity planning model has discrete variables and is an optimization problem. The general model assumes capacity as a discrete figure using a steady stream of queuing approximations with capacity costs set to constraints equaling service levels desired. This model can be modified easily to accommodate capacity increases as well as capacity decreases.

Six queuing stations were used for the blood bank example:

1. Registration,
2. Fill-out forms,
3. Donor screening,
4. Preparation for donating blood,
5. Donate blood, and
6. Canteen.

At each of the six activity stations, arrival rate was approximated, server (whether nurse, donor, or staff) was listed, and capacity was defined as limited or unlimited. Nurse and staff salaries and donation stations are constraints. Capacity costs versus average time in the blood bank (in minutes) were calculated in graphic form. As average patient time in the system is reduced, capacity costs increase at an increasing rate.

Patient flow for the HMO clinic was determined as

1. Sign in and waiting room,
2. Nurse's station,
3. Examining room,
4. Lab, x-ray, and
5. Check out.

At each of the five activity stations, arrival rate per day was collected along with the standard deviation, server (whether nurse, physician, or staff) was listed and capacity was defined as limited. Also, minimum, average, median, maximum, and standard deviation of times for the clinics in minutes were calculated for each activity station. Specific data was not available in the study due to confidentiality.

The queuing network model captured the probabilistic nature of health care systems and measured customer service levels within optimization outlines. The multi-period extension of the model gives recommendations for the size of capacity and timing requirements. This type of extension is important when the number of patients are not expected to be constant over the planning time span.

"What if" analyses can be used to assist administrators in understanding the tradeoff between capacity and patient time in the system. The model can be used to define the stop point in patient time beyond which further reductions become prohibitively expensive or impractical. A nice feature of the model is that mean and standard deviation of the arrival and service rates are all that is required for input. The model is very flexible for capacity planning. The model can also be used in non-health care settings.

8.2 ADMINISTRATIVE DAYS IN HOSPITALS

The days a patient spends in a hospital waiting for the provision of extended care service such as a nursing home, social support services, or home health care services are referred to as administrative days. Prediction of the length and frequency of these administrative days would provide very valuable information which could be used to improve the performance of a hospital. A model was developed using a queuing analytic approach to describe the process by which patients await placement after receiving acute care. Model results were compared with data gathered from various hospitals in New York State.

Researchers Elliott N. Weiss of the University of Virginia, Charlottesville, Virginia and John O. McClain of Cornell University, Ithaca, New York (1987), developed a model of the queuing system for patients waiting for placement in an extended care facility and presented both analytical and empirical results to support their findings. Weiss and McClain presented alternative analytical models for the queuing situation and then analyzed data from seven upstate New York hospitals in order to estimate and validate the model.

A model was developed of a single acute care facility which is only applicable when there is one acute care facility and one extended care facility. The model depicted three categories of patients:

1. patients for whom extended care is not necessary,
2. patients who will need extended care but whose status is currently acute, and
3. patients who are "backed up" or blocked by lack of extended care facilities.

The research concentrated on a solution for a single-facility model and considered only those patients who would eventually require extended care.

Assumptions were made for the single facility model. Alternate level care (ALC) patients arrive randomly and depart according to a rate that is dependent on the extended care placement process of the hospital. Departures of ALC patients were based on the total system placement process. The model showed that the placement success rate per patient increased as the census increased. This can also be interpreted: As the census increases, there is more pressure placed on the discharge planning staff to place patients and less pressure when the ALC census is low. The researchers called this the restoring force model. As the census increased the placement rate per patient increased and vice versa.

The results of the data analysis concluded that the census of ALC patients could be modeled using a very simple, service rate model. There were some slightly underestimated patient distributions which were likely a result of the variability of the census distribution. The underestimated results were not enough to reject the hypothesis.

As the cost of holding patients in an acute care facility rise and the population of the United States continues to age, ALC patients who are backed up in acute care facilities will be responsible for elevated health care costs which in turn will be passed on to the consumer. Use of these models can give hospital decision makers information with which to evaluate a cost-benefit tradeoff which will lead to improved quality of care measures. These models can assist hospital management in the controlling of the discharge planning staff budget and resource allocation. These models can also be used to evaluate the feasibility of increasing the number of extended care facilities (ECF) to handle the backed up patients in hospitals. To fully utilize the models the authors suggest that additional models be created to discover the relationship between the discharge planning staffing levels and budget to the ALC patient days and quality of care.

8.3   EVALUATION OF OUTPATIENT APPOINTMENT SCHEDULING

An important problem service oriented organizations face is the question of how long to schedule appointments and the sequencing of these appointments so that the service provided is the most efficient. Physician's offices, medical clinics, and other health service offices run into this dilemma every day. They want to keep provider idle time to a minimum, minimize client waiting time, and provide time slots for emergencies that may arise.

Kenneth J. Klassen and Thomas R. Rohleder of University of Calgary in Alberta, Canada (1996), used prior research results, interviews with medical clinic receptionists, and a computer simulation to research the appointment problem. Their research tested the relations of the different causal factors and evaluated the best way to set up the appointment schedule for the outpatient scheduling problem.

The researchers first interviewed medical office personnel who deal with this issue every day. They found that, on average, scheduled medical appointments last about 10 minutes. Clients are also scheduled based on a number of other criteria, such as medical problem, age, and past experience. They found that client characteristics were not a factor when scheduling. Clinic personnel all felt that, on average, appointments were slightly longer than the slots that were assigned to them. Normally, clients are labeled as regular, urgent, or serious. The serious clients were not included in the study because these clients were often told to go straight to the hospital. On average, the clinics left 1 to 3 empty slots for urgent calls per half day session.

The vehicle for this study was a computer simulation model. It was assumed that clients arrive punctually, clients are served only once per visit, each session was independent, and a few slots had to be left for emergencies. The simulated half day sessions consisted of 3-1/2 hours of scheduling time, and ten minute appointment times were used. To generate the number of calls per session a distribution with the mean of two was used.

The goal of the research was to minimize the weighted average of client waiting time and service provider idle time. The simulation model allowed the weights to be varied. The location of the urgent slots in the schedule was extensively evaluated. It was decided that they must be positioned towards the end of each session so that urgent calls that come in late have a better chance of being serviced during the session. There were 21 time slots during each session and the urgent call slots were positioned at locations 10 to 12. Statistical tests confirmed that the selected location was best.

The next step was to compare all the scheduling rules with statistical tests and select the best one. Two specific rules tested were the high variance start (HVS) rule and the low variance start (LVS) rule. The HVS rule requires that the first high variance client who calls is scheduled in slot 1, the second in slot 2, and so on. The first low variance client who calls is scheduled in the last slot (slot 21), the second low variance to call is scheduled in slot 20, and so on. The LVS rule is the opposite of the HVS rule. It was found that generally the LVS rule worked best.

Clients are developing higher expectations of medical service providers while competition between these service providers is intensifying. People have low tolerance for long waiting times. They do not want to sit and wait in a doctor's office for hours just because the doctor does not want idle time and his schedule is double booked. The research by Klassen and Rohleder tells us a lot about this issue, but, as they are quick to point out, there is a lot of room left in this area to still be researched.

8.4   NURSE STAFFING LEVELS
IN U.S. HOSPITALS

Cost containment pressures have given rise to the redesign and restructuring of the clinical workforce. Public concern regarding the effect of this on the quality of patient care has been recognized, yet little evaluation has been conducted regarding the effect of restructuring on the quality of care. Very few studies have addressed the contribution of nurse staffing to the frequency of avoidable adverse events. In the fourth quarter 1998 issue of *Image*, Christine Kovner of New York University, and J. Gergen of the Agency for Health Policy and Research (AHCPR), describe the results of one such study.

Description of Study

The authors conducted a survey with 1993 discharge data from the Nationwide Inpatient Sample (NIS) from the AHCPR, then matched this data by using hospital identification numbers from American Hospital Association (AHA) annual survey data from the same year. A probability sample was used from all community hospitals in ten geographically dispersed states. Related hospital characteristics were controlled. NIS discharge data was used to extract hospital level indicators of adverse events. Hospital level variables included teaching status, ownership, bed size, hospital resources, region, relationship with a managed care organization, and nurse staffing. Nurse staffing was determined by the number of full time employee (FTE) registered nurses (RNs) working in the hospital and in the outpatient departments per adjusted patient day.

The relationship between nurse staffing and nurse-sensitive events versus non-nurse-sensitive events was empirically tested. The adverse events were further delineated according to quality indicators developed by the Healthcare Cost and Utilization Project-3. Patients at risk for these complications due to their major diagnostic category, as opposed to the event being an avoidable surgical complication, were eliminated. Adverse nurse-sensitive events included in the study were as follows:

1. thrombosis or pulmonary embolism after major surgery,
2. thrombosis or pulmonary embolism after an invasive vascular procedure,
3. urinary tract infection after major surgery,
4. pneumonia after major surgery, and
5. pneumonia after an invasive vascular procedure.

Non-nurse sensitive indicators were:

1. pulmonary compromise after major surgery, including pulmonary edema and respiratory failure, for example,
2. acute myocardial infarction after major surgery,
3. gastrointestinal hemorrhage after major surgery,
4. mechanical complications because of device, implant, or graft (excluding organ transplant).

Results

Significant inverse relationships were found to exist between nurse staffing and the following post operative adverse events: urinary tract infections, pneumonia, thrombosis, and pulmonary compromise after major surgery. Additionally, hospital level variables also were significantly related to these events, as follows: Large hospitals had significantly lower urinary tract infection rates than small hospitals, and large and medium size hospitals had significantly higher pulmonary compromise rates. Not-for-profit hospitals, as well as hospitals with nursing school affiliation, had significantly lower post-operative pneumonia and pulmonary compromise. Also, hospitals with FTE nurse practitioners did not have significant relationships with adverse events, although hospitals with physician assistants had higher rates of pneumonia and thrombosis after surgery. Hospitals with a higher percentage of Medicare patients had higher rates of urinary tract infections.

The relationship between these adverse events and nurse staffing is clinically important. For example, an increase of 0.5 RN hours per patient day is associated with a decrease of 0.16 urinary tract infections per 100 surgical patients at risk. Accordingly, an increase of 0.5 RN hours per patient day is related to a 4.2 percent decrease in pneumonia, a 2.6 percent decrease in thrombosis, and a 1.8 percent decrease in pulmonary compromise after surgery.

Implications Health Care Organizations

When considering staff cuts and restructuring, the strong relationship between nurse staffing and avoidable adverse events in this study should be considered. It is cost-effective to decrease adverse events. And, of course, it is good for patients and for the organization's reputation. For example, hospital acquired pneumonia accounts for up to 20 percent of all hospital acquired infections in hospitalized patients. Should nurse staffing be increased? What is the maximum acceptable level of adverse events? These questions must be addressed by health care executives, managers, and policy makers. Just as with any clinical intervention, the effect of clinical reorganization on patient care must continue to be examined.

8.5 HIGH-PERFORMING PROJECT MANAGEMENT ORGANIZATIONS

Development of new pharmaceutical products involves coordinated activities between many different functions within a company over a period of many years. The success of a project is based on significant investment in research and development (R&D) and long-term planning. Drug development activities outsourced to contract organizations continue to increase and cover more areas of R&D. Outsourcing is used to cover gaps in capacity, increase a company's skill base, and control costs. However, outsourcing activities require additional emphasis on the company's management of the overall development project. Completion and external pressure to bring new products to the market faster continues to increase in the pharmaceutical industry. In order to gain a competitive advantage to do so, and more cost effectively, companies need to refine their project management processes to ensure resources are adequately assigned to the most promising projects, and non-viable projects are terminated as early in the process as possible. Due to the complexity and multi-functional nature of pharmaceutical development, various approaches to pharmaceutical project management have evolved. The relative effectiveness of different approaches on project performance is largely unknown.

Dr. Randolph Case, Assistant Professor, Operations and Strategic Management, Boston College, Boston, MA (1998), was chosen as the lead investigator responsible for designing and implementing the study, sponsored by the Pharmaceutical Research and Manufacturers Association (PhRMA), a trade organization representing R&D-based pharmaceutical companies.

The study was designed to determine how various approaches to pharmaceutical project management impact organizational performance and to identify critical success factors for managing projects. Because the success or failure of a project is typically due to the characteristics of the drug itself, rather than the manner in which the project was managed, it was recognized that success or failure would not be appropriate outcomes for the study. Also, as the pharmaceutical development process spans many years, the project management style over the course of a particular project is likely to change several times. Therefore, the study was designed to gauge the effectiveness of various approaches in real time, i.e., to measure organizational performance reflecting the project management approach at the time the data for the study were gathered. The study therefore collected data on theories in practice, meaning, that the most effective project management approaches were the ones currently in practice, or in the minds of the scientists and managers currently working in the industry.

The study involved twenty U.S.-based pharmaceutical development organizations of various sizes. The study was organized into two parts. Part I consisted of in-person interviews of at least four managers at each of the firms. These four people consisted of: a leader of a development project ream, the head of project management, a functional department head, and the top executive in R&D. These interviews largely consisted of asking the respondents to describe how project management in their firm had changed in the past year, or, needed changing and why.

The main observations collected in Part I were used to design Part II of the study. Part II consisted of a written questionnaire completed by the project leader of each existing development project within each firm. The questionnaire measured six dimensions of project-organization integration, and measured project performance. In addition, Part II consisted of a telephone interview with a member of senior R&D management in each firm. In these telephone interviews, the executive assessed the effectiveness of each of the development projects, and the overall effectiveness of the firm's project management efforts.

The study data were analyzed using multiple regression in which a number of project management variables reflecting a dimension of project-organization integration were regressed separately against two different measures of project performance. For resource allocation it was found that priority for resources and team size were significantly related to a performance measure. This suggested that the highest performing projects are those that have been given a priority position among the other projects in the portfolio, along with sizable teams. For commitment, it was found that team members' emotional attachment to the project, and matrix-structured teams, in which the members do not report primarily to the project leader, but to their functional department (or both), are clearly associated with project effectiveness.

Higher performing projects were ones in which the project was related to an area of technical competence by the firm, and in cases where the project was not wholly owned by the firm (e.g., ventures and co-development projects). Outsourcing parts of projects did not undermine project performance.

It was also found that project leaders should be in a physically proximate location with the team members, but at a distance from functional departments. Also, project performance is typically higher when decisions are influenced more by the team members than by functional or senior management.

High performing teams are given focused attention and resources to provide priority status and financial backing, but also space and independence as well. Team members should maintain a link with their functional departments to provide technical expertise, but be more emotionally tied to the project. With a project being less integrated with the organization, the firm can be more objective on it, and therefore place more focus on priority projects or terminate less promising projects with fewer political ramifications. Disintegration with the functional departments also pushes more authority onto the team, which makes the team more motivated to push the project along.

The research done by this study provides valuable insights into critical success factors in creating high performing project teams. The main dimension studied was the degree in which the project team is integrated with the rest of the organization. From this information, companies can gauge their project management efforts versus performance, and implement changes within their operational structure to incorporate the factors found in this study to be associated with high performing teams.

8.6 WORK TEAMS AND MANUFACTURING PERFORMANCE

Implementation of work teams generally improves performance in manufacturing. This is the overall conclusion of Banker, Field, Schroeder, and Sinha (1996) after their study of an electric motor assembly plant. Manufacturing operations that implement a work team philosophy can expect quality to increase and can expect productivity levels to rise leading to a real transformation in the workplace.

One of the key findings of the study point to the fact that the level of improvement in both quality and productivity are tied to the level of cohesiveness and cooperation within the work team. This is dependent on each individual work team. In the same environment some teams will excel far beyond others troubled by conflict and friction.

The study was performed over a 21-month period during which a work team philosophy was implemented. During the first four months of the study the work teams did not exist. During the remaining 17 months the work teams were organized and the teams were observed to evaluate their performance. The manufacturing operation being studied included four production lines. There was no cross training or job rotation either between any of the four production lines, nor within any of the four teams.

The teams were made up of the production workers, a production engineer, the production planner, and the plant manager. A facilitator was assigned to the teams. This was the same person for all four teams. The facilitator's role is to organize and train the teams. The facilitator was not a team member; a leader of each team was chosen from within the team.

One team was made up of highly-trained production workers who were machinists. These workers generally had higher seniority and had a much higher level of cohesion from the beginning of the study. This team performed better and had larger gains in both labor productivity and in quality than any of the other teams. One team in particular had a great deal of internal conflict. There were still gains in both productivity and quality but the difference made by the conflict was noticeable in the results of the study.

Another key of the study was the evolution of the tasks the teams took on as they matured. There was a noticeable shift from individual to group-level issues. The tasks being assigned also shifted from being assigned to the production engineer to being assigned individual team members or to the team as a whole.

The study is not without its shortcomings, however. The research team points out the lack of a control plant where no work teams were introduced. Therefore, it appears that additional empirical study of this subject matter is warranted. The described study is a good start at examining an issue which prior to this study had not really been tested through scientific means.

8.7   HIGH PERFORMANCE WORK SYSTEMS

With the recent positive attention given to High Performance Work Systems (HPWS), can it be assumed that constant levels of success can be achieved throughout the U.S.? Through a critical analysis of the literature available, the systems effectiveness of HPWS was rated. In addition, certain recommendations were made to those considering implementing a HPWS.

Gerard F. Farias and Arup Varma (1998) conducted this analysis to first examine whether these HPWS were indeed effective and secondly, to prescribe the most effective use of these systems. Since so much information is available about the effectiveness of HPWS, Farias and Varma felt that by sifting through this documentation they could get a better understanding of implementing and maintaining High Performance Work Systems.

In an attempt to better understand the working of HPWS, the researchers set out to define it. Prior research offered them insight into the workings of HPWS from which they drew their own conclusions. Also the emergence of reports showing the results of HPWS aided them in developing a universal theme.

The researchers examined two separate surveys of Fortune 1000 companies and their use of these HPWS. These studies showed an increasing trend towards employee involvement in Total Quality Management (TQM) practices. Another study illustrated how these same companies were forced to modify their human resource practices in order to implement HPWS. This was important in identifying the overall cost of using these systems. The researchers also discovered that HPWS were easier to implement in new work units rather than in existing ones. This is important to keep in mind when considering using a HPWS. Yet another study assessed the state of HPWS in service industries. This study found that although significant improvements in operational and financial performance were noted, there was little impact on the outcomes.

In spite of these positive results, the researchers took a holistic approach to this issue and identified certain reasons this study may not show the complete picture. First, they believe that the negative outcomes of HPWS may be overlooked in favor of keeping their image positive. It is also important to note that this reporting bias has also ignored the debate over whether the systems can support themselves in the long run.

While the researchers admit that it is difficult to find two identical designs within corporate America, making it difficult to defend comparisons and generalizations, they have identified several factors organizations planning to adopt HPWS must consider. First, they identify change within organizations as frail and often subject to derailment. HPWS must be implemented carefully. Secondly, companies must adopt a HPWS that is capable of changing with the organization. Third, companies must be patient with HPWS, because often their benefits take a while to emerge.

These findings are of great importance to organizations. The researchers have shown that HPWS are not a fad, and that their use can usually assure success. They point out that this is not a universal theory and has to be applied to each situation differently. This is important for companies attempting to use a HPWS. Finally, HPWS have been shown to be progressive and productive additions to organizations.

8.8   PURCHASING PRACTICES BY JUST-IN-TIME FIRMS

A sharp increase in competition over the last three decades has led to a significant increase in material outsourcing. A typical total product cost consists of nearly 55 percent of outsourced materials. Firms are demanding top quality when it comes to the purchased materials that go into their final product. Due to this, firms are redesigning their purchasing processes and re-evaluating their relationships with their suppliers. The explosion of just-in-time (JIT) production procedures has also helped to bring about this evolution in purchasing.

The research conducted by Vonderembse, Tracy, Tan, and Bardy (1995) focused on the changes that purchasing is undergoing. Two thousand members of the Midwest region of the National Association of Purchasing Managers were sent a questionnaire. The questionnaire contained 268 questions. The questionnaire was based on a five-point Likert scale. Four areas were targeted: 1. criteria for supplier selection, 2. changes in purchasing practices, 3. shifts in the levels of interaction with other functional areas and with vendors, and 4. strategic partnerships. The study split the participants into two groups, JIT users and non-JIT users.

Results of the study revealed that JIT producers put a greater emphasis on product performance and product quality. The study also found that firms are reducing the number of trucking companies that they use for delivering their purchased materials. This is a result of firms attempting to lower their freight rates by encouraging carriers to increase their loads. Lead times were also found to be decreasing. In addition, the study concluded that JIT users showed higher interaction rates than non-JIT users between inventory management, outside transport, and engineering. However, with respect to interaction involving purchasing and vending, JIT and non-JIT users both showed an increase.

The last part of the study found that suppliers are being reduced by both JIT and non-JIT firms. The remaining JIT suppliers are making greater strides to improve quality and reduce costs. The study found that overall, purchasing is becoming a critical factor in the competitive global market. JIT firms are benefiting more from these purchasing improvements than non-JIT firms. In general, JIT firms are in a better position to meet the current demands of the market.

REFERENCES

Banker, R. D., Field, J. M., Schroeder, R. G., & Sinha, K. K. (1996). Impact of work teams on manufacturing performance: A longitudinal field study. *Academy of Management Journal, 39*(4), 867-890.

Bretthauer K. M., & Cote, M. J. (1998). A model for planning resource requirements in health care organizations. *Decision Sciences, 29*(1), 243-270.

Case, R. J. (1998). The structure of high-performance project management organizations. *Drug Information Journal, 32,* 577-607.

Farias, G. F., & Varma, A. (1998). Research update: High performance work systems: What we know and what we need to know. *Decision Sciences Journal, 21*(2), 50-54.

Klassen, K. J., & Rohleder, T. R. (1996). Scheduling outpatient appointments in a dynamic environment. *Journal of Operations Management, 14,* 83-101.

Kovner, C., & Gergen, P. J. (1998). Nurse staffing levels and adverse events following surgery in U.S. hospitals. *Image: Journal of Nursing Scholarships, 30*(4), 315-321.

Vonderembse, M., Tracy, M., Tan, C. L., & Bardi, E. J. (1995). Current purchasing practices and JIT: Some of the effects on inbound logistics. *International Journal of Physical Distribution and Logistics Management, 25*(3), 33-48.

Weiss, E. N., & McClain, J. O. (1987). Administrative days in acute care facilities: A queuing-analytic approach. *Operations Research, 35*(1), 35-44.

CHAPTER 9

INFORMATICS AND HEALTH CARE

This chapter addresses the issue of informatics in health care. Implementation of informatics in the health care system has been slow, fragmented, expensive, and tedious. It will take considerably more time, effort, and financial investment before the health system is able to fully benefit from the information technology that is available now and will be in the future.

The first study looks at HMO data systems and access to health care. The study used data from the National Health Interview Survey (NHIS). The survey is a survey of households that reaches the majority of the population. The study revealed that although HMO members have lower hospital utilization rates, the information systems utilized by HMOs leave much to be desired. In general, HMO databases contain little information on both their membership and services provided. Little information flows from providers such as physicians and hospitals back to the HMOs. Hence the connection between providers and HMOs needs to be strengthened before the HMOs can be useful sources of patient information.

The second study is one on retrieving and transferring embodied data with implications for management of interdependence within organizations. An example of embodied data is a problem encountered by a patient during a doctor visit. The problem occurred at an earlier time but is not

Proven Solutions for Improving Health and Lowering Health Care Costs, pages 127–140.
Copyright © 2003 by Information Age Publishing, Inc.
All rights of reproduction in any form reserved.
ISBN: 1-59311-000-6 (paper), 1-59311-001-4 (cloth)

diagnosed until later during a routine office visit. In the paper's case the focus of the study was manufactured assembly but the analogy to a patient as an assembly is not far-fetched. Information on a patient's health can be collected at a variety of locations such as in a doctor's office, an emergency room office, a hospital, an ambulance, a rehabilitation facility, a pharmacy, etc. All the information needs to be deposited into one location: the patient's file. To do this is still a major problem—a problem addressed in this study.

The third study describes a system for monitoring and evaluating the long term care of the elderly and disabled. The purpose of the system is to have a reliable and valuable database of the health care and health needs of the elderly. The system provides management information that is useful for managing the health care needs and resources that would not be available from other sources. The data are easy to analyze and the data collection does not cause an extra burden on the health care system.

The fourth study explores the effects of reminders for outpatient influenza immunizations. The purpose of the study is to evaluate the influence of computer-based reminders about the influenza vaccine on the behavior of individual clinicians at each clinical opportunity. The study was done at a large internal medicine clinic with 34 clinicians taking part in the study. About half used computer-based records (CPR) and the other half used paper records (PR) for their respective patients. The results of the study showed that patients who had CPRs had increases in compliance rates for influenza immunizations from 40% to 68%, while the patients who were managed with PRs had increases in compliance rates for influenza immunization from 28% to 31%. The positive increase among the CPR user group reflects how the use of a CPR can improve the degree to which guidelines are followed.

The fifth study explores the effects of decision aids on health center site locations. Eighteen professionals consisting of accountants and consultants were used in the study. The problem they were assigned consisted of determining optimal site locations for six proposed 24-hour health care centers in a metropolitan area. Each professional was given access to the same demographic data. Some of the professionals were also given access to a spreadsheet decision aid, while the remainder only had use of a calculator. The research showed that the professionals with decision aids took over 50% more time to reach a decision compared with those who did not have access to the decision aid. Unfortunately what could not be determined was how good the decisions of each group were. Those using the decision aids clearly could evaluate more alternatives and in more detail. For investment decisions such as in this case the more alternatives that are explored the better is usually the final decision.

The sixth study describes an empirical test of the strategic grid model of information systems (IS) planning, a common planning tool used by informatics specialists. For this study 27 government agencies were required to follow the strategic grid model of IS planning, while 22 other agencies could select a method of planning selected by them. The results obtained were equivocal. Some of the mandated planning approaches were not appropriate for some agencies, thus creating more problems than solutions. The implications of the study indicate that a mandated single approach for IS planning is not appropriate for all situations.

The seventh and final study identifies the drivers of customer satisfaction for software products. Seven key determinants of customer satisfaction with software products and service support were identified. The seven factors are reliability, capability, usability, installability, maintain ability, performance, and documentation. The factors that influence customer satisfaction vary across product groups, and customer segments. The three most important factors are capability, usability, and performance in their influence on customer satisfaction. Hence software producers should poll their potential customers to determine which factors are the most important to them, and then provide software that focuses on the indicated factors.

In this chapter we have addressed a number of papers which looked at a cross-section of informatics problems in the health field. Much work still needs to be done in the development and implementation of informatics systems to improve the information recording, handling, and reporting of health data.

9.1 DATA SYSTEMS AND ACCESS TO CARE

This study looks at the current status of HMO data sets and their applicability to population studies of access to care. The authors looked at the content of HMO reports, such as the completeness of the reports, their processing and reporting. In general, the majority of HMO's give reporting information on the scope of services provided to their members, but are unable to give an individual patient report on the services to the individual.

The researcher of this study is Raymond Fink (1998). With the rising importance of HMOs in our health care system, it is important to measure the members' accessibility of care. The researcher measures accessibility by the number of contacts with various providers as well as if contact was made with the provider, including the frequency and variety of contacts. These include measures of utilization commonly used in health services research, including rates of utilizers, mean number of services provided, hospital admissions, and length of stay. The primary sources of this data include surveys of the population regarding the scope of health services received, the patient's medical records, electronic medical or billing records, and hospital discharge reports.

The population study used as data is the National Health Interview Survey (NHIS). This survey is a household survey that reaches a majority of the population. The reason such a survey is used is based on the fact that most health insurance plans lack sufficient identification information to permit linkages between demographic information and service utilization, particularly outpatient care.

The study found that there were lower hospital utilization rates among HMOs as compared to other health care delivery systems. This information is substantiated in both admission reports in addition to the length of stay. The study also critiques the data systems of HMOs. Their observation are as follows: In general HMOs are not able to develop reports on specific members in regards to services rendered. In addition, there may be concerns about incomplete service counts due to provider failure to submit encounter information, reports are largely anecdotal, and the magnitude of the problem unknown. Also, the HMO databases are rather limited. The databases contain little information on both their membership and the services provided. Finally, there is little information regarding the accuracy of the data. They do not know much about the information received from the providers. Also, there could be errors in the processing of the information received.

Overall, this study has many implications for business. This could help HMOs to look into their database systems to see if better data collection is possible. The information supplied in these databases can be very helpful for many others outside the organization, such as hospitals, the government and individual providers. By providing more accurate and extensive information, HMOs can produce individual reports on their patients. This information can include accessibility of health care and the medical services received. This information can also help to streamline their organizational knowledge into one system.

9.2   COLLECTION OF EMBODIED DATA

An example of embodied data in manufacturing is a defect in a component which is discovered during the assembly process. The defect occurred upstream but is discovered during the downstream assembly activity.

It can be costly for an organization that utilizes sequential processes, when downstream operators discover errors in the upstream activity. Not enough emphasis is currently being placed on direct communication between downstream and upstream to facilitate information that will help benefit the upstream process. Several means for managing organizations to reduce such costly coordination problems have been suggested, but each has limited applicability and each can be expensive.

Researcher Andrew King of the Stern School of Business, New York University (1994), performed case studies of eight manufacturers of printed circuits. He felt that this was a good choice because the industry has an excellent domain in which to explore embodied data in sequential tasks. In this industry King chose to investigate information transfer between the upstream process and downstream process.

King surveyed upstream managers of these manufacturers to discover what they felt were their most important process changes, what rate of importance was the department that initiated these changes, and what were the relative effects of each process change. King also interviewed at least two downstream managers and two staff members at each manufacturer. When the data was collected a point scale was given to each construct. The mean, standard deviation, and correlation of variables were used in a regression analysis. This analysis was then used to prove or disprove the six hypotheses of the paper.

The first hypothesis states that the more downstream processes are sensitive to upstream process variation, the more often they will retrieve and transfer information to the upstream process. This was proved through the finding that as more sensitive equipment was used, the more frequently information was passed. The data did not prove the second hypothesis. Neither the formal education of the upstream manager nor his previous experience in a production job provided any additional explanatory power. The data did support hypothesis 3. Physical distance seems to decrease the frequency with which upstream personnel pass helpful information to the downstream engineering manager. The data seems to suggest that intimacy is indeed important to upstream information transfer. Likewise, the data weakly supports hypothesis 4 that states joint participation on teams and task forces seem to support communication of useful information.

The data did not support hypotheses 5a or 5b. Incentives to improve plant performance or cooperate with other departments did not add explanatory power to the model. Thus, the data provided no evidence that management rewards significantly influenced the acquisition and transfer of information. The data partially supported hypothesis 6, in which downstream engineering managers reported that they more often received useful information from upstream personnel when upstream activities had relatively less access to monetary resources from top management.

This case points out that in some cases the negative effects of interdependence can be lessened by an increase in the retrieval and transfer of embodied data. This data also suggests that in some circumstances, an organization should not seek to reduce interdependence but to increase it. What is clear from the data is that the retrieval and transfer of embodied data can help improve the interdependence process that manufacturers use.

9.3   MONITORING AND EVALUATING LONG-TERM CARE

The ASIM monitoring system was developed in 1984 and established in 1987 as a method of monitoring the flow of clients to and from the health care system and between different cells of the system. Each cell measures a combination of a level of care and a measure of need. The regular staff of the care unit where the client is registered gathers the data for the yearly survey, which takes a picture of the status of clients in the system on a given day. This survey is repeated on an annual basis. The data that are gathered in the survey are:

1.   the client's national registration number,
2.   the present health care system unit,
3.   any application to another level of care,
4.   appropriate level of care and,
5.   amount of assistance, social environment, and disability of the client.

Specific criteria were developed to assist the staff member in determining the disability level of the client. However, no such criteria were developed for the appropriate level of care; this determination is left to the professional judgement of the staff member.

This study looks at the survey data to determine if it is complete, reliable, and valid. The goal of the study is to determine if the ASIM is meeting the needs of health system management and if it is a useful tool for monitoring and evaluating the long-term care of the elderly. Dr. Lagergren (1993) studied data from the ASIM system from the period of 1984 to 1990.

Methods Completeness is a measure to see if all of the clients in the system were included in the surveys and if all health system units delivered the entry forms. Because of the fact that there is not a database of the total number of clients in the health care system at any one time, it is not possible to verify the completeness directly. However, by comparing the survey data from one year to the next one can identify clients—by the national registration number—that are in one survey and not in another without a corresponding admission or discharge record. Through this method some uncounted clients were identified. If a client was found to be missing from a survey, clarification was requested from the health care system unit and a corresponding correction was made to the survey data. However, if a client were missed by two succeeding surveys, that client would remain uncounted for the purposes of this research.

Dr. Lagergren also measured the reliability of the data. This was measured by locating and examining involuntary double assessments of the same client. These duplications were detected by examining the national registration numbers in a survey. To measure the validity, the duplicate entries were compared to see if the same answers were given.

The validity of the data is a measure of how the data reflect the factors that the health system management requires to manage the system effectively. As the purpose of the ASIM system is to measure the needs of the clients against the availability of resources; the validity was measured by comparing appropriate level of care with the allowance for home help and home health care in domiciliary care and sheltered housing. It was also measured by comparing the level of disability with the allotted hours of home help and home health care.

Results: As was mentioned in the methods section, there is no accurate way to directly measure the completeness of the data. However, using the indirect method described in the Methods section, it was estimated that less than one percent of clients were missing entirely from the survey during the period between 1984 and 1987. After 1987 is was not possible to track missing clients as accurately due to the fact that the discharge and admittance registrations were no longer taken. However, it was judged that only a small percentage of clients were still missing. While these small percentages will not have an adverse affect on the results of the data analysis, the author noted that it is troubling to observe that people in need of care may not be receiving it.

The reliability of the data was measured using the duplicate registrations. When duplicate registrations were examined, uniformity of assessment between the first and second registration appears low, with exact matches being .59 and close matches being .78. The uniformity is higher when only double registrations from the same health system unit are compared. Under this comparison, exact matches are .77 and close matches are .90. The reliability of the five different disability measures was also tested using the involuntary double registrations. The results of this test are better than the test of uniformity of assessment, with results between .73 and .84 for exact matches, and increasing .97 to .99 if close matches are included. Again, the results worsen if double registrations across units are included. A systematic basis in rating the appropriate level of care appears when the double registrations are examined based on the level of care the health care system unit provides. Analysis of the data shows that three of the five variables describing disability are strongly correlated to the appropriate level of care. These variables are functional disability, incontinence, and dementia. Mobility, disability, and insecurity were not as highly correlated. It is important to note that the reliability of the data may be questioned due to the fact that some health system unit staff members may have biased the data in order to achieve some end unrelated to the actual situation of the client, such as showing a need for increased staffing at the unit.

The validity of the appropriate level of care as a measure of need was studied by comparing the correlation between these two factors. The results show that as the level of need increases, so do the allotted hours of care. Analysis shows that there is high correlation between the level of disability and the level of care, especially with functional disability, incontinence and dementia. Therefore, these measures are a valid way to assess the need for care.

Implications

While the data gathered in the ASIM system is not as scientifically developed and gathered as it would be in a research project, the ASIM system does give management information that is useful for managing the health care needs and resources—data that would not be available from other sources. The data are easy to analyze and its collection does not cause an extra burden on the health care system. The conclusion is drawn that the ASIM is an effective tool for the management of a health care system.

9.4   EFFECTS OF REMINDERS FOR OUTPATIENT INFLUENZA IMMUNIZATIONS

The computer-based patient record (CPR) is a valuable tool whose reminders can help clinicians act on each opportunity to provide preventive health services and to promote healthy behavior. When CPR users open the chart of a patient eligible for a recommended intervention, rule-based clinical reminders appear, informing the clinician of alerts concerning the patient's problems, medications, allergies, procedures, health maintenance, and laboratory results. Managed care plans often require provider organizations to report how well their practitioners comply with clinical guidelines.

Although influenza vaccination is strongly recommended to people aged 65 and above, actual vaccination rates are between 45 and 58 percent. Immunized patients have been shown to have approximately half the death rates, half the hospitalization rates, and half the hospital costs of non-immunized patients. Computer-based reminder systems can increase clinicians' rates of compliance, especially in preventive health maintenance interventions.

Description of study

The research, described in the March/April issue of the *Journal of the American Medical Informatics Association,* was conducted by P. Tang of Northwestern University and Northwestern Memorial Hospital in Chicago, and by M. LaRosa, C. Newcomb, and S. Gorden, all of Northwestern Memorial Hospital (1999). The purpose of the study was to evaluate the influence of computer-based reminders about the influenza vaccine on the behavior of individual clinicians at each clinical opportunity.

This was a prospective study conducted at a large internal medicine clinic at an academic center with 34 clinicians. Approximately one half of the clinicians used a previously implemented CPR (CPR users), while the other clinicians used traditional paper records (PR users). Clinicians were assessed in terms of what actions they took when presented with the opportunity to follow the influenza guideline. Guideline compliance was achieved by performing one of the following four actions:

1. ordering the vaccine,
2. documenting that counseling was performed,
3. documenting that the vaccine was offered but the patient declined, or
4. documenting that the patient had already received the vaccine elsewhere.

After the patient received or declined the vaccine, he or she was considered ineligible for the remainder of that year's influenza season. If the patient had only received counseling, then the patient remained eligible for the vaccination.

All patients aged 65 and older who had one or more non-acute clinic visits during the influenza season from 1995-1998 were included. The CPR user group had a total of 1,536 patient visits by influenza guideline eligible patients for the time period studied, while the PR user group had 1,581. No statistical differences between groups existed in terms of the distribution of chronic medical conditions. Data was abstracted from the medical records and imported to SPSS for analysis.

Results

Compliance rates with the influenza vaccination guidelines for the CPR users for 1995-1998 increased from 40.1% to 68.2%. PR user compliance rates for the same period was 27.9% to 30.6%.

Implications

The positive increase among the CPR user group reflects how the use of a CPR can improve the degree to which guidelines are followed. Improved documentation is rising in importance both for quality reporting and for reimbursement compliance. Many health plans now request that clinicians document counseling about various preventive measures and treatments. The CPR automates the capture of accurate information which can be used to evaluate the effects of interventions designed to help improve compliance with guidelines at every opportunity.

9.5   EFFECTS OF DECISION AIDS ON HEALTH CENTER SITE LOCATION PLANNING

Past research on decision aids concentrated on one of the following areas:

1.   Studies that examined whether the use of decision aids increased decision quality or some work performance measure;
2.   Studies geared towards identifying the most effective design characteristics and parameters of decision aids, and
3.   Studies that identified characteristics of decision makers and their interaction with decision aids.

Research had been lacking in the area of evaluating the effect of decision aids on the problem-solving process.

Researchers Jane M. Mackay of Texas Christian University, and Steve H. Barr and Marilyn G. Kletke, both of the Oklahoma State University (1992), conducted a research study consisting of nine accountants and nine health care planning consultants. The purpose of their research was to study whether decision aids facilitated decision makers in certain areas of the problem-solving process.

The researchers broke the problem-solving process down into three stages:

1.   problem presentations,
2.   problem representation, and
3.   problem solution, in order to measure the results of their research.

The problem presentation stage consisted of only one step, which they called problem finding. The problem representation stage consisted of the following steps: problem formulation, idea generation, and idea evaluation and integration. The problem solution stage consisted of the following steps: idea execution, solution identification, and retrospective evaluation.

The task assigned to the subjects was to determine optimal site locations for six proposed 24-hour health care centers in metropolitan areas. Each subject was given access to the same demographic data. Some of the subjects were given access to a decision aid, Lotus 1-2-3, while others were not.

The subjects who were proficient in Lotus 1-2-3 were labeled as experts in decision aids; otherwise they were labeled as novices. Subjects were also labeled as experts or novices based on their work experience with regards to the assigned task. In all there were six subject classifications:

1. task novices/decision aid novices,
2. task novices/decision aid experts,
3. task experts/decision aid novices,
4. task experts/decision aid experts,
5. task novices with no decision aid access, and
6. task experts with no decision aid access.

The researchers identified four areas of measurement to track:

1. time to reach the final solution,
2. time spent in each of the problem-solving steps,
3. number of actions in each of the problem-solving steps, and
4. time spent to identify potential solutions.

The method used to measure the subjects in these areas was verbal protocol analysis. Verbal protocol analysis consists of the subjects talking out loud about what they are doing, as they are doing it. The researchers recorded these conversations as well as video taping the subjects.

The research showed that subjects using decision aids took over fifty percent longer to reach a final decision compared to subject that did not use a decision aid. The research also showed that the time spent in the various problem-solving steps varied significantly between decision aided, and non-decision aided groups. Subjects using Lotus 1-2-3 spent more time in the problem finding and problem solution steps, because Lotus 1-2-3 gave them the ability to examine a larger number of alternatives. Another conclusion from the study was that the interaction between task familiarity and decision aid familiarity plays a role in the time spent in various steps of the problem-solving process.

Research of this nature can be used to help developers of decision aids. Decision aid software developers could use this research data to examine how people are using decision aids, and how long they spend in each step of the problem-solving processes. This data could be used to identify certain areas that users spend a lot of time on. The software developers could then determine if the user spends a lot of time in these areas, because certain aspects of their software are not easy to use, or because these areas are of a significant importance to the user. Using this information, decision aid software developers could enhance aspects of their software that are weak or limited in nature.

9.6   AN EVALUATION OF THE STRATEGIC-GRID INFORMATION SYSTEMS PLANNING MODEL

In this paper questions are asked regarding information systems planning. Can any single planning approach suit all organization's needs? Contingency models of information systems planning indicate that this is not the case. These researchers intend to evaluate this further in order to add to the little empirical research that already exists.

Researchers Semi Tukana, a management information systems specialist with the Fiji Development Bank, and Ron Weber, with the Department of Commerce at the University of Queensland (1996), used a strategic-grid model to study information systems planning problems encountered by forty-nine government agencies.

For this study, twenty-seven agencies were required to follow a planning approach best suited to organizations that had a high level of dependence on both their existing and proposed systems. It was predicted that agencies not having these characteristics would encounter the most problems with the approach. The remaining twenty-two agencies could choose their own planning approach.

The group using their own planning approach were studied to determine whether the problems encountered by the first group could be attributed to the mandated approach. In addition, the problems encountered by the group using the standard approach were studied to determine the causes and the degrees of these problems. The researchers used the strategic-grid model for these purposes. They also attempted to investigate how organizational learning impacts planning behaviors, and to determine the types of information systems planning problems that diffuse through organizations and those that remain localized.

Overall, the researchers state that the empirical results they obtained were equivocal. Some results indicated that more planning problems were encountered by agencies in which the mandated approach was not appropriate to their position in the strategic grid. Other results, however, were not supportive of this proposition. The researchers feel that more work needs to be undertaken to evaluate the predictive and explanatory power of contingency models of information systems planning. Also, they believe more rigorous theories of information systems planning behaviors need to be developed. They also found that the instruments needed to measure these behaviors need to be improved.

This study's implications for business need to be further developed. It seems, however, that a mandated single approach to information systems planning would not be appropriate for all businesses. More work and definitive measures should be undertaken in order to provide statistical proof of this theory. The real implications on business at this point, are that each organization must find an information systems planning strategy that accommodates their particular needs and suits their characteristics.

9.7 SOURCES OF CUSTOMER SATISFACTION FOR SOFTWARE PRODUCTS

In this paper, seven key determinants of customer satisfaction with software products and service support are identified. The analysis provides important information to the program designers and marketing managers of a software company to identify how their software should be designed to satisfy customers.

The researchers, Sunder Kekre, Mayuram S. Krishnan, and Kannan Srinivasan (1995), identified seven determinants consisting of reliability, capability, usability, installability, maintainability, performance, and documentation. However, the factors that influence the satisfaction of customers vary across product groups. For example, performance is the key factor for network products. The relative importance of the factors also varies across customer segments. For example, usability is the critical factor for the novice users. However, capability, usability, and performance are the three most important factors that influence satisfaction. If any one of the seven factors improves, it will yield a shift in the customer's satisfaction level.

A key limitation of the data used is that the pool was limited to current IBM customers. Since the dissatisfied customers are not likely to remain as IBM's customers, the use of only IBM data could be a big flaw of the research. This research still needs broader and deeper research to get more reliable results. The sample should be enlarged to include both IBM and non-IBM customers.

Improving customer satisfaction has become a big issue in the software industry. Understanding the drivers of customer satisfaction is the critical first step toward customer satisfaction. The paper provides important information for making design and service support choices for software products.

REFERENCES

Fink, R. (1998). HMO data systems in population studies of access to care. *Health Services Research, 33*(3), 741-760.

Kekre, S., Krishnan, M. S., & Srinivasan, K. (1995). Drivers of customer satisfaction for software products: Implications for design and service support. *Management Science,* **41**(9), 1456-1469.

King, A. (1994). Retrieving and transferring embodied data: Implications for the management of interdependence within organizations. *Management Science, 45*(7), 918-934.

Lagergren, M. (1993). ASIM: A system for monitoring and evaluating the long-term care of the elderly and disabled. *Health Services Research, 28*(1), 27-45.

Mackay, J. M., Barr, S. H., & Kletke, M. G. (1992). An empirical investigation of the effects of decision aids on problem solving processes. *Decision Sciences, 23*(3), 648-672.

Tang, P. C., LaRosa, M. P., Newcomb, C., & Gorden, S. M. (1999). Measuring the effects of reminders for outpatient influenza immunizations at the point of clinical opportunity. *Journal of the American Medical Informatics Association, 6*(2), 115-121.

Tukana, S., & Weber, R. (1996). An empirical test of the strategic-grid model of information systems planning. *Decision Sciences Journal, 27*(4), 735-765.

CHAPTER 10

HUMAN RESOURCE MANAGEMENT IN HEALTH SYSTEMS

This chapter addresses issues in managing the work force in health care institutions. Although the studies reported on are not necessarily in the health sector, the issues addressed are generic and apply to all job settings.

The first study is concerned with group absence behavior and employees' perceptions of absence standards, and their concurrent absence behavior. The research showed that there are significant differences between groups in their perception of absence standards, and absenteeism is correlated with absence standards perceptions. The implication for management is to ensure that absence standards are maintained at a high level across the various organizational units.

The second study reports on the types of employer-employee relationships that prevail in organizations. Four types of relationships were evaluated ranging from strict payment for services performed to overinvestment by the employer in the employee through training, further career opportunities, and broad-ranging reward systems. Nearly 1000 employees in 85 different jobs employed by 10 organizations were analyzed. The results

Proven Solutions for Improving Health and Lowering Health Care Costs, pages 141–154.
Copyright © 2003 by Information Age Publishing, Inc.
All rights of reproduction in any form reserved.
ISBN: 1-59311-000-6 (paper), 1-59311-001-4 (cloth)

showed that the higher the investment by the employer in the employee the better the employee performance and employee attitude.

The third study addresses the complex issue of how to reward chief executive officers (CEOs) of corporations to insure that they make decisions that are in the interest of the owners, and as a result in the interest of the long term health of the corporation. The results of the study showed that CEOs who invested the generated cash from operations in promising new investments generated better performance for their corporations than CEOs who conserved the generated cash flows. The performance measure consisted of the performance of the shareholder value of the firm investigated.

The fourth study was an investigation of gender differences in behavior, demographics, and productivity of middle managers. The study environment was the banking industry. The study showed that although men and women eventually can reach the same positions, the women have significantly lower earnings when productivity, demographics, and behavioral differences are controlled. Despite this wage gap, the study showed that important salary factors are education, experience, and employment restrictions as opposed to outright gender bias.

The fifth study addressed the interesting question of a male ceiling for traditionally female jobs. A group of nearly 200 mature business students (average age was 29 years) were asked to evaluate two male and two female applicants for two positions in an educational institution. The material available for evaluation of the applicants was biased in terms of qualification for the respective jobs. The results of the study showed that some rankers selected for management a less qualified female instead of a more qualified male when the job was traditionally female.

The sixth study reports on whether job satisfaction is related to intelligence. The results are interesting and need to be studied carefully. In general, intelligence is positively related to job satisfaction because more intelligent people get more interesting and complex jobs. But intelligence is negatively associated with satisfaction when complexity is held constant. These results are interesting for employers. To maintain or increase job satisfaction, employees should be placed in jobs that are aligned with their intelligence levels.

The seventh and last study explored the relationship between social identity and minority workers' health. The study's database consisted of 88 participants from four different organizations. The results of the study showed that minority workers' social relationships help them cope with work-related stress, which can lower the instances of health problems.

The seven studies summarized above provide several instances of scientifically proven approaches management can use to improve the job satisfaction and other job attributes which will improve the overall performance of the affected organizations.

10.1 ABSENCE BEHAVIOR FOLLOWS ABSENCE STANDARDS

Employee absenteeism is a major concern for management in an organization. Absenteeism can cause an overall decrease in productivity, which can cost an organization large amounts of money every year. In the past, absenteeism research has been characterized by a focus on the behavior and attitudes of individuals. However, in the 1980s research investigated the potential impact of an organization's social context on employees' perceptions of absence standards and their concurrent absence behavior.

Researchers Steven E. Markham and Gail H. McKee (1995) defined two measures of absence standards and examined how those constructs operated at three different levels of analysis:

1. individuals,
2. supervisory groups, and
3. plants.

Using techniques for analyzing multi-level data, Markham and McKee's experiment is based around the concept of absence climate as a social interaction mechanism. Climate is defined as the common practices, procedures, and beliefs followed in an organization. More specifically, a salient absence climate is one in which there is agreement within groups about absence beliefs and attendance practices.

The researchers asserted that the supervisory group to which an employee belongs would affect a variety of absence climate indicators, including, but not restricted to, internal and external absence standards. Furthermore, when information is unclear to members of a social unit they will interact to make sense of the information. Citing another reference, the researchers point out that given continuously changing workplaces without some informational framework, all organizational actions and outcomes are inherently ambiguous. It follows that work groups become an important vehicle for their members' efforts to make sense of a work environment. The researchers point out that supervisory groups will serve as anchors for shared similarity in perceptions and behavior.

The first group-level hypothesis the researchers formulated posits that there will be differences between supervisory groups in terms of actual absence behavior. The researchers state that if absence does not differ by supervisory groups, it is difficult to argue that absence standards are, in fact, correlated with group differences in absence behavior.

The second hypothesis asserts that there will be significant differences between supervisory groups in their members' perceived external standards of absence. Additionally, supervisory groups sharing low external standards (i.e., management is viewed as accepting many absences) will have, on average, more absence incidents than those with high standards.

The third hypothesis asserts these same principles applied to external standards.

The fourth hypothesis addresses supervisors' views of internal and external standards. This hypothesis asserts that supervisors' views of internal and external standards will predict their group's levels of absence incidents.

The research locations used were five garment factories in the Virginia-North Carolina region. All five factories belonged to the same company. Confidential questionnaires were administered to all 1,216 employees. The sample size was reduced to 1,019 due to incomplete questionnaires. Employees were asked to provide their names so their responses could be matched against their absenteeism records. It is important to note that surveys were administered to regular employees as well as supervisors.

The company's attendance policy cited perfect attendance as the goal. This policy was conveyed to employees both orally and through written materials. Furthermore, at each plant employees could be dismissed for excessive absence. Employees were not paid when they were absent and more than 90% of the respondents were paid on a piecework basis.

The dependent variable for the experiment was the attendance records. A full year's attendance records for all individuals were collected covering the six months prior to the survey and the six months after it. The questionnaire did not appear to cause a substantial fluctuation in absence.

The independent variables included the questions used to measure absence standards. To measure the external managerial standard, the question was: What do you think management's goal for absenteeism is for you? The second variable, internal personal standard, was measured by the following question: IN YOUR VIEW, what is an acceptable level of absenteeism here?

The results of the questionnaire confirmed the first three hypotheses. The research confirmed that there actually are group differences in absence behavior. This is central to the argument of saliency. The research also supported the hypothesis that there will be significant differences between groups in their perception of management's goal for absence and that the correlation of group averages on the absence frequency measure agrees with group averages on the managerial standard measure.

The first part of hypothesis 4 was supported but the second part was not. Supervisors' views of external managerial standards did *not* predict their group's absences; however, the supervisors' views of *internal personal standards did* significantly predict their group's absences.

The implications of this study for business are significant. Because as a group may affect the absence standards of its members, it is important to initially address absence standards strategically and in such a way that promotes high group absence standards in various supervisory groups. This research also draws attention to the fact that absence climate may not be a single effect pervading an entire organization; rather, units within an organization may have different climates (and absence rates).

10.2   PERFORMANCE AND THE EMPLOYER - EMPLOYEE RELATIONSHIP

Employees performed better on core tasks, demonstrated more citizenship behavior, and expressed a higher level of effective commitment to an employer when they worked in an Overinvestment (by the employer) employee-organization relationship or Mutual Investment relationship than when they worked in a Quasi-Spot-Contract or Underinvestment relationship. An employee-organization relationship includes the employer's expectations about specific contributions that it desires from employees, and the inducements that it uses to effect the desired contributions. The focus of the study came from the perspective of the employer since this is where most of the recent changes have taken place in terms of downsizing, consolidation and the like, as well as the fact that although negotiations do occur, it is the employer who defines the bulk of the terms of employment contracts.

The researchers of the study are Anne S. Tsui, Jone L. Pearce, and Lyman W. Porter of the University of California at Irvine, and Angela M. Tripoli of University College Dublin (1997).

Four employer-defined employee-organization relationship approaches were studied. The first two involved balanced exchanges between the employer and employee.

1. *Quasi-Spot Contract*—This resembles a purely economic exchange. The employer offers short term economic inducements in exchange for a well defined contribution by the employee. Neither party expects any inducements beyond those specified. The balance is that it is short term and closed ended for both parties. An example would be between a brokerage firm and a stockbroker.
2. *Mutual Investment*—A willingness expressed by the employee to learn firm-specific skills that are not easily transferable to another company. The employee trusts that this will be reciprocated over the long term. It is balanced in the sense that it is an open ended, long-term investment by both parties.

There are also two un-balanced employee-organization relationships. These include:

1. *Underinvestment*—Here the employee is expected to undertake broad, open ended obligations, while the employer reciprocates

with short term and specified monetary rewards with no commitment to a long-term relationship or investment in the employee's training or career.

2. *Overinvestment*—Represents a relationship that consists of the employees doing well specified set of job-focused activities. The employer offers open-ended and broad-ranging rewards, including training and further career opportunities.

The study focused on companies in competitive industries. Ten companies, in five industries, with at least 1,000 employees were identified. Testing was done at the individual job level, utilizing only permanent employees. Union employees were excluded. In the end, 976 employees, in 85 different jobs, from the 10 companies were analyzed. The demographic characteristics included age, company tenure, education, gender, and race.

Written surveys were used to collect data. Confidentiality was assured to all. Supervisors gave information pertaining to that employee's employee-organization relationship, and rated their employee's performance. Employees provided ratings for themselves, and their co-workers. The measures that resulted from this data collection included the employee-organization relationship, employee performance, and attitude measures. These measures were applied to seven hypotheses.

The statistical analyses showed that both Mutual Investment and Overinvestment were associated with higher level of performance and more favorable attitudes toward the work place, with Mutual Investment being the overall best approach. However, the results also showed that the employee-organization relationship needs to be chosen carefully. The approach taken needs to match both the job and the employees being managed. Even more challenging is specifying performance outputs while at the same time protecting long term organizational interests. The study suggests that offering open-ended inducements and a high level of social exchange to employees is more important than the balance in the exchange.

So, while money is not the motivator that many would think that it is, this study shows that employees seem to flourish in an environment of commitment versus control. While financial gains will be part of the equation, there is a great deal to say for the old adage that, "You have to like what you are doing."

10.3   CEO COMPENSATION AND THE INVESTMENT BEHAVIOR

The main issue that this article (McConaughy & Mishra, 1997) focuses on is how shareholders can control managers when it comes to using free cash flow in the best interest of the company. The researchers believe that when free cash flow is available, the use of incentive-based compensation (for managers) becomes an internal control strategy for the shareholders. The firms that are likely to struggle from this situation the most are the high cash flow and high growth firms, due to the fact that their assets are not as easily monitored. The main study focus of this article is to provide insight into the underinvestment problem (managers not taking advantage of new opportunities) and whether the growth, size, and cash flow variables of the firm play a role in the issue.

The research sample consists of 430 firms from a study by Jensen and Murphy in 1990. The data shows the pay performance sensitivity of a dollar change in the chief executive officer's (CEO's) pay per $1,000 change in shareholder wealth. The pay performance sensitivity was further broken down into short-term compensation, which includes salary and bonuses, and long-term sensitivity, which includes stock options. The control period for the 430 firms is between 1974 and 1988 and contains the data found in the Forbes executive compensation surveys. The test period is from 1989 to 1993 and reviews the effect of increasing stock option incentives during this time. The study was further broken down by one digit SIC codes and the industries with fewer than 10 firms were deleted from the study, which left 395 firms in the sample.

The main parameter that McConaughy and Mishra studied during the test period was the abnormal return of the firms. Abnormal return is a risk adjusted measure that takes the total return and subtracts off the expected return for the firm. The return data was drawn from the daily stock market data files.

The objective of the test was to determine under which conditions of growth and cash flow, increasing pay performance sensitivity, is associated with improved firm performance. The authors believe pay performance sensitivity to be dependent upon size, growth opportunities, leverage, and cash flows of the firm.

The theories behind this study indicate that the managers will not always invest in positive net present value (NPV) projects due to the feeling that the shareholders, being diversified, are risk neutral. Also if the managers are risk neutral and the firm is one of high growth the shareholders have no control mechanisms to ensure that all the positive opportunities are being invested. Pay performance incentives for managers will act as this control mechanism especially when the incentives are tied to the long-term performance of the firm in terms of stock options. This is why, as studies have shown, CEOs of growth firms receive more of their compensation in terms of long-term incentives. The theories predict that firms with high cash flow will end up with lower positive abnormal returns, while firms with lower cash flow will experience more positive abnormal returns due to their investments in opportunistic situations. The researchers also predicted that increasing pay performance sensitivity in firms with abundant growth opportunities is associated with higher firm performance.

The results of the study indicate that the firms that chose higher cash flows are associated with lower performance. This is explained by claiming that the excess cash flow results from the failure to invest in positive NPV opportunities.

Another important finding of the study is that for high growth firms, long-term pay performance sensitivity is associated with higher firm performance. Short-term pay incentives on the other hand, show no statistical evidence of increasing the firm performance.

The major implication presented of this study is the validation of long-term pay performance compensation in high growth firms. It also shows the significance of cash flow and how excess cash flow usually leads to lower firm performance.

10.4   GENDER DIFFERENCES IN PROMOTION AND COMPENSATION OF MIDDLE MANAGERS

The focus on this study centered around the perceived gender wage gap between males and females at the middle manager position in the banking industry. The authors concentrated on various characteristics such as behavior, demographics, and productivity to help explain the wage differences.

Statistics show that in the banking industry 84 percent of employees, 46 percent of the bank managers, and only 4 percent of senior executives are women.

The researchers who conducted the study, Linda Martin and Sandra Morgan (1995), began by surveying 106 middle bank managers of which 25 were men and 81 were women. The sample was represented by managers who were seen by their supervisors as up and coming, and represented no significant sample bias with regards to position level, education, or experience.

The survey asked the managers questions that would provide insight into demographic, behavior, and productivity differences between the two genders. The demographic measures used were such characteristics as age and marital status. Productivity factors were experience, education, and the number of promotions; and the behavioral factor was attribution for success.

There have been many theories and studies on the wage gap between genders that have provided the researchers with initial hypotheses. For example, human capital studies have shown that the difference between earnings is a result of a weaker attachment to the workforce or a lower investment in education by the part of the women. There are conflicting studies however that show women are being held to higher promotion standards and receive less on-the-job training than their male counter-parts. A study in 1982 found that for men and women in the same position, the women were promoted much more often to get there. Still other researchers found that the differences in gender behavior and attitudes is the reason for the wage gap. Finally, the attribution theory proposes that men view their success is attributable to their skill and hard work, while women view their success as luck. These are some of the theories that the researchers were trying to test.

The research found that in the demographic category, the female mid-dle managers were older, more likely to be married, and had more chil-dren living at home. The study showed no significant difference in the initial age of hiring between the men and women.

Productivity results from the study show that the women in the sample are less likely to have a college degree, but that women have attended sig-nificantly more training courses provided by the bank. It also shows that women had to work on average 10.5 years in the banking industry to achieve middle manager status, while it took the men only 6 years. During their rise to middle manager status, the women received 2.9 promotions compared to the men's 1.6 promotions. The research also found that women on average have significantly more restrictions on their careers than do men (due to spousal employment, child raising, etc.). What these productivity factors indicate is that although men and women start their banking career at the same age, women will be older by the time they reach middle management.

With regards to behavioral status, the study found that the men attribute their success to luck much more frequently than do the women, which is an opposite finding from previous studies. The desire or aspiration to high levels within the bank was virtually the same for both genders.

The major implications of this study are that although men and women eventually can reach the same positions, the women have significantly reduced earnings when productivity, demographic, and behavioral differ-ences are controlled. Despite this wage gap, the study did show that impor-tant salary factors are education, experience, and employment restrictions as opposed to outright gender bias. The researches were successful in attributing the wage difference (at least in middle managers in the bank-ing industry) to factors that are rational and controllable.

10.5 A CEILING FOR MALES IN TRADITIONALLY FEMALE JOBS?

A fairly well-qualified group of business students, most were employed and over half had management experience, were asked to rank hypothetical male and female job applicants for top- and middle-level management positions in a traditionally female job. The job consisted of Dean (top-level) and Coordinator (mid-level) in a School of Social Work.

The study was completed by Leanne E. Atwater and David D. Van Fleet of Arizona State University West in Phoenix, Arizona (1997). The students used in this study also came from this university.

The student rankers were 191 business students about equally divided between men and women. Most were employed, over half had management experience and their average age was 29 years. The student rankers were asked to review two packets of material; each packet included materials describing job characteristics about two male and two female applicants for the Dean position and the Coordinator position respectively. In each scenario, one of the males and one of the females was clearly under-qualified relative to the other two candidates. The qualified male and female each currently held the same job and the male was noticeably more qualified than the female. The research team purposely biased the qualification in favor of the gender opposite the gender-typed job. In other words, the male was more qualified for both the top-level and mid-level positions. With this method, if a female were selected or given a higher salary, it would be clear that the decision was not based on the applicants' qualifications but rather in spite of them.

Over one-fourth of the student rankers selected a less-qualified female over a more qualified male for both the Dean's job and the Coordinator's job. Additionally, those student rankers with management experience tended to make decisions favoring the less-qualified female more than those without management experience. The results suggest that males may suffer from discrimination in traditionally female jobs similar to that faced by females in traditionally male jobs.

In summary, the most interesting result of the study was the tendency for some student rankers to select for management a less qualified female rather than a more qualified male when the job was traditionally female. It appears that a lack of consistency between an applicant's gender type and the gender type of the job is a basis for discrimination against males in "female" jobs. That less-qualified females were selected over their better qualified male competition is troublesome given the recent attention paid to workplace diversity and equal employment opportunity. It appears possible that so much attention has been devoted to discrimination against women and minorities that the issue of equal opportunity does not yet embrace men as well.

10.6   IS JOB SATISFACTION DIRECTLY RELATED TO INTELLIGENCE?

A person's level of intelligence is strongly correlated to many outcomes in a person's life. Is intelligence also a predictor of job satisfaction? The problem is that while much research has been done on the situational and motivational effects on job satisfaction, very little research has looked at how large, or how little, a role a person's level of intelligence plays in job satisfaction. Is there a relation between wisdom and happiness?

Yoav Ganzach, from Tel Aviv University (1998), and his colleagues wanted to see if they could find the answer to this question. The relationship between intelligence and satisfaction was analyzed on the basis of a model in which intelligence has a direct negative effect on job satisfaction, an indirect positive effect, mediated by job complexity, and an interactive effect with job complexity. Background variables, such as level of education, were also taken into account.

The first hypothesis states that intelligent people desire more complex work and consequently are dissatisfied with their jobs. This is revealed when job complexity is held constant. Hypothesis 2 states that intelligent people find complex work and are more satisfied with their jobs. This is an indirect positive effect, mediated by job complexity, revealed when job complexity is varied. The third hypothesis states that job complexity moderates the direct negative effect of intelligence on job satisfaction. The higher the complexity of a person's job, the less negative the relationship between intelligence and satisfaction.

The data were taken from the National Longitudinal Survey of Youth with a sample of 12,686 Americans with no oversampling of the economically disadvantaged born between 1957 and 1964. Several variables were used, including a number of control variables such as sex, age, ethnic origin, etc. Intelligence was scored by summing the results of the four sections of the Armed Forces Qualifying Test: arithmetic reasoning, paragraph comprehension, word knowledge, and math knowledge. Occupation was determined from respondents' descriptions. Job complexity was measured using two scales. The first was derived from the Job Diagnostics Index and looked at degree to which they worked with others, autonomy, feedback, opportunities for friendship, opportunities to complete tasks, task identity, and task variety. The second measure was "DOT complexity." It is a summary index of the characteristics of occupations evaluated by job analysts. These include data complexity, educational preparation, abstraction, and degree of verbal and numerical aptitudes. One last variable was global job satisfaction which measured the degree to which participants liked their jobs. These variables were regressed to find the results.

The results were fairly consistent with the hypotheses. Intelligence is positively related to job satisfaction because more intelligent people get more interesting and complex jobs. But intelligence is associated negatively with satisfaction when complexity is held constant. The negative direct effect of intelligence is mediated by job complexity. There is no simple answer to the question about the relationship between intelligence and job satisfaction. The answer depends on the question if this relationship is analyzed between jobs or within jobs, and if it depends on the jobs being analyzed.

These results can be applied in businesses in several ways. First, employers must determine what type of tasks and what type workers they have. Where the tasks are fairly routine, and the individual is intelligent, it would be wise to either increase the difficulty level of tasks, give a variety of tasks, or perhaps move the individual to a position of higher responsibility. This will keep the employee more satisfied with his job and will consequently cut down on turnover. Where the tasks are highly complex, a change in jobs is not necessary to keep job satisfaction high for highly intelligent people.

10.7 SOCIAL RELATIONSHIP AND MINORITY WORKERS' HEALTH

There has been recent attention to the effect of work-related stress on an individual's health. It has been shown that social relationships may help people deal with stressful events in the workplace. For minorities, this might be a problem, since they typically do not make up the majority of the workforce. Because of their racial identity, they may have fewer social relationships at work and therefore are less resistant to work-related stress. There has been a lack of research on the effect of stress on minorities. This study concentrated on how minority workers' social relationships at work and social-behavioral tendencies influence their health.

Researchers Keith James, Chris Lovato, and Gillian Khoo from Colorado State University (1994) received funding from The Graduate College at Colorado State University to research these issues. They examined six variables as potential correlates of minority workers' health. The variables were:

1. levels of self-esteem (ethnic-group-based),
2. levels of collective esteem (ethnic-group-based),
3. levels of perceived prejudice experienced on the job,
4. levels of perceived discrimination experienced on the job,
5. perceived differences in values between minorities and supervisors, and between minorities and peers (assessed separately), and
6. individual expressiveness.

The researchers formulated eight different hypotheses based on the six variables of interest.

The study consisted of eighty-eight participants from four different organizations. Two of the companies were private manufacturing firms, one was a unit of State government, and one was a private social service agency. Sixty or 68 percent of the participants were women and 28 (32 percent) were men. The population was made up of 64 percent Mexican American, 18.1percent African American, 10 percent Asian American, 3.4

percent Native American, and 4.5 percent of mixed heritage. The participants were paid $7.50 each.

Paper and pencil measures were used for each of the correlates of health. Prejudice and discrimination consisted of sixteen items, each with a seven-point scale. The self-esteem measures included seventeen items with a five-point scale, while the collective esteem inventory used four items, each with a seven-point scale. The value differences correlate measured three items with a seven-point scale. Expressiveness was measured using fifteen verbal tendencies and fifteen non-verbal tendencies.

The researchers also looked at blood pressure for an objective measure in addition to the self-reports on health, which was taken using an illness checklist. The control variables were age, weight, and type of organization.

Participants were divided into two groups; one group consisted of individuals who reported high blood pressure and the other group did not report high blood pressure. The group that reported high blood pressure had higher readings (average reading of 211.63) than the second group (average reading 184.50), which proves the validity of using the blood pressure measures and illness checklists. Regression analyses were run for the blood pressure readings and for the illness checklist. The blood pressure regression shows that value differences between a participant and his/her supervisor, expressiveness, prejudice-discrimination, and self-esteem correlates had statistically significant effects on the minority worker's health.

The results of the study indicate that minority workers' social relationships help them cope with work-related stress, which can lower the instances of health problems. Minority workers perceive discrimination, prejudice, and value differences between them and their supervisors as major sources of stress.

In the mid-1980s, General Motors spent close to $800 million a year on health-related costs for their employees. Cardiovascular problems were the most costly. It is apparent that companies today need to concentrate and come up with solutions for these types of problems. Organizations must create an atmosphere that welcomes and respects workplace diversity.

REFERENCES

Atwater, L. E., & Van Fleet, D. D. (1997). Another ceiling? Can males compete for traditionally female jobs? *Journal of Management, 23*(6), 603-626.

Ganzach, Y. (1998). Intelligence and job satisfaction. *Academy of Management Journal, 41*(5), 526-539.

James, K., Lovato, C., & Khoo, G. (1994). Social identity correlates of minority workers' health. *Academy of Management Journal, 37*(2), 383-396.

Markham, S. E., & McKee, G. H. (1995). Group absence behavior and standards: A multilevel analysis. *Academy of Management Journal, 38*(4), 1174-1190.

Martin, L. R., & Morgan, S. (1995). Middle managers in banking: An investigation of gender differences in behavior, demographics, and productivity. *Quarterly Journal of Business and Economics, 34,* 55-69.

McConaughy, D. L., & Mishra, C. S. (1997). The role of performance-based compensation in reducing the underinvestment problem. *Quarterly Journal of Business and Economics, 36,* 25-38.

Tsui, A. S., Pearce, J. L., Porter, L. W., & Tripoli, A. M. (1997). Alternative approaches to the employee-organization relationship: Does investment in employees pay off? *Academy of Management Journal, 40*(5), 1089-1121.

CHAPTER 11

ORGANIZATIONAL BEHAVIOR IN HEALTH SYSTEMS

This chapter covers the behavior and dynamics in organizations. The chapter is related to the human resource management chapter but focuses more on organizational issues versus employee issues. However, a significant overlap exists between this and the human resource chapter.

The first study covers the effects of job demands in a hospital setting. The job category focused on was the registered nurses group. The research showed that as the workload increased for those who had low control in their jobs, job satisfaction decreased significantly. For those nurses who had high levels of job control their job satisfaction remained fairly steady.

The second study studied career developments in the health care industry focusing on female executives. The specific areas looked at was the use of mentors for both male and female managers. The results showed that women did not experience more difficulty in finding mentors than men. There was some evidence that women tended to have more women mentors while few men had women as mentors.

The third study explored the effects of organizational behavior modification on task performance in service versus manufacturing organizations. The results show that there are differences between manufacturing and service organizations when applying operant learning and reinforcement

Proven Solutions for Improving Health and Lowering Health Care Costs, pages 155–168.
Copyright © 2003 by Information Age Publishing, Inc.
All rights of reproduction in any form reserved.
ISBN: 1-59311-000-6 (paper), 1-59311-001-4 (cloth)

theory to improving task performance. The results show that financial, non-financial, social, and combinations of reinforcements have a significant effect in both manufacturing and service organizations. In service organizations, financial reinforcement produced the strongest effect, but non-financial incentives produce essentially the same results as financial incentives.

The fourth study describes how research shows that effects of different types of leadership styles are mitigated by humor. A sample of top management team members was surveyed to determine the use of humor in their interactions with subordinates. The results indicated that the use of humor for some leadership styles will reduce the negative effects of the chosen leadership style. The positive effects of humor minimizes the effects of avoidance behaviors displayed by laissez-faire leadership. It appears that humor creates a climate that allows subordinates to feel better about their work environment despite their dissatisfaction with a chosen leadership style.

The fifth study explores the effects of gender on leader emergence. The study was performed on groups of students working as groups on structured case analysis projects outside of class hours. These projects forced the students to work together and observe each other. Since no group leaders were appointed leadership had to emerge within each group. Following the group projects the students were surveyed for their observations on leadership emergence. The results of the study revealed that masculinity was correlated with self-perceived and group-perceived leader emergence. It was also found that gender role is a better predictor than just gender. Hence women who had masculine tendencies were more likely to emerge as leaders than androgenous (displaying characteristics of both sexes) men.

The sixth study was based on research on trust and distrust in organizations. Researchers found that trust and distrust are not reciprocal of each other, but are separate but linked dimensions. The implications of the study point to a need for individuals in organizations to trust their fellow staff members, but at the same time ensure that proper monitoring is in place of what all employees are doing. A classic example is the need for control systems in organizations. These control systems are able to function in a culture of trust.

The seventh and final study addresses work-related stress resulting from contact with AIDS patients. The study explores if a nurse's exposure to AIDS patients as part of the job is positively associated with distress (negative mood) at work. The research showed that there was indeed a correlation between exposure to AIDS and negative mood. Negative mood was weakest when organizational support and social support were high. The results suggest that health care organizations need to provide adequate support to nurses who deal with AIDS patients.

In this chapter we have addressed issues relating to the interface between employees and organizations. In this day and age the welfare of the employee is increasingly recognized as a key to obtaining maximum effectiveness from employees and maintaining satisfied employees is one way to achieving the maximum effectiveness.

11.1   EFFECTS OF JOB DEMANDS IN A HOSPITAL SETTING

What connection exists between job stress, and jobs that are high in work demands and low in controllability? Also, does the stress one encounters in the work place carry over into one's personal life, after one leaves work? These are the basic issues that are covered in this paper.

Researchers Marilyn L. Fox, Deborah J. Dwyer, and Daniel C. Ganster (1993) tested the job demands—job control model. The underlying principle of the job demands—job control model is that job stress, which results in mental and physical health problems, occurs in occupations where the employee faces high demands and low control in their everyday work. The researchers tested this model using a group of 136 registered nurses as their subjects.

The following areas of measurement were used in this study to test the job demands—job control model: work demands, job control, overall job satisfaction, and physiological outcomes. Both objective and subjective work demand measures were used. The objective work demands included: patient load, patient contact hours as a percentage of total work time, and the number of deaths witnessed on the job over the past year. Subjective work demand measures were obtained by having the nurses complete a questionnaire using a 7-item scale measuring the amount and pace of their work. Control measurements were obtained via the nurses completing a 22-item scale questionnaire designed to capture the nurses' perceptions of the amount of control they have at work. The nurses were asked how much control they had in the following areas of their jobs: variety of tasks performed, the order in which they could perform their work tasks, their work pace, work procedures and policies, and arrangement of their work environments. A 17-item scale questionnaire was used to measure the nurses' overall satisfaction, and inquired about such illnesses as insomnia, headaches, and upset stomachs that the nurses may encounter. Physiological outcomes were measured using arterial blood pressure readings and salivary cortisol readings. Arterial blood pressure is one of the risk factors leading to cardiovascular disease. Salivary cortisol readings are an indication of ineffective coping, and when an individual is having a hard time meeting the physical demands placed upon them.

The nurses, who were from the same hospital but from several different departments, took their blood pressure readings and saliva collections for three straight days. Saliva was collected right after waking up, once at work, and once two to three hours after leaving work. Blood pressure readings were taken right after waking up, three different times at work, and three different times after leaving work. The saliva collections were less frequent than the blood pressure readings, due to the extensive nature of the lab tests required to obtain cortisol levels from the saliva samples. The research study extended over a two month period, and the nurses were picked at random for their three day study period in order to eliminate bias that could occur due to outside variables that could influence specific departments in the short run.

The research showed that as the workload increased for those who had low control in their jobs, job satisfaction decreased significantly. This was not true for those who had high levels of control in their jobs. Another finding was that cortisol levels and blood pressure, both at work and at home, increased as the workload increased for those with low levels of control in their jobs. This was not true for those with high levels of control in their jobs. The research found that as the number of stress events increased for those with low levels of job control, job satisfaction decreased significantly, but remained fairly steady for those who had high levels of job control. All of the above findings supported the job demands—job control theory. The one finding that did not support the theory was that as the number of deaths increased, job satisfaction did not significantly decrease for those with low levels of job control, but it did for those with high levels of job control.

One of the trends in the health care industry has been towards health maintenance organizations (HMOs) and controlling health insurance costs. In order to achieve this goal, health care organizations have been increasing workloads of their employees. This research would suggest that if health care workers were not given more control in their jobs, then their mental and physical health, as well as their job satisfaction would be adversely affected. Managers in other professions could use this research model and apply it to their specific areas also. If they have subordinates with heavy workloads, and low levels of control in their jobs, the manager may consider giving them more flexibility in how they perform their jobs.

11.2 GENDER AND CAREER DEVELOPMENT IN THE HEALTH CARE INDUSTRY

Does cross-gender mentoring on the career development of executives in the health care industry have a positive influence on the career paths of female executives and their chances for promotion in their organizations and are the relationships influenced by gender differences? Research has shown that mentoring relationships offer reciprocal benefits for the mentor and the protégé, they provide a support mechanism for individuals and promote cultural diversity within the organization. Mentors can provide valuable psychosocial functions as well as a foundation and potential ladder for career advancement. However, there are some variables, such as gender differences, that could present obstacles for some in developing these relationships and benefiting from them.

Data for this study was collected using a questionnaire that addressed four main hypotheses and was given to 1,680 members of the American College of Health Executives. A Kruskal-Wallis test was used to analyze the data and to formulate results on demographic, organizational variables, and mentor functions for both male and female managers. The questionnaire addressed various stereotypes and preconceived notions about women in the health care industry and their experiences with mentoring relationships. Little research has been done in this area but some research has shown significant differences in the mentoring relationships between genders.

The researchers Walsh and Borkowski (1999) tested several hypotheses. The first hypothesis in the study questioned whether women would experience more difficulty in accessing mentors in the health care industry. In the past women were seen as tokens in organizations and were not excluded socially but were treated unequally and not given access to the same career opportunities that men had available to them. The second hypothesis questioned whether organizational policies and reward systems would limit access to mentors for female managers in the health care industry. It was felt that the absence of a formal rewards system would deter managers from participating in a mentor program with women or take the time to help them advance in their careers. The third hypothesis addressed intimacy concerns and questioned whether issues like this would limit social interactions in cross-gender mentoring relationships. This is a sensitive issue and has gotten a lot of publicity over the past few years mainly because of all of the sexual harassment cases that have gotten public exposure and the bad press that has planted a seed in the minds of many people about the risks of being involved in relationships with women. The last hypothesis in the study questioned whether mentor functions and behaviors would differ in relationship with male and female managers. This question related to the previous issue of intimacy and the notion that these issues could have caused people to alter their behaviors and become ultra sensitive towards females just to protect themselves against any potentially dangerous situations or predicaments.

The results of the study produced some very interesting findings that refuted many stereotypes and findings that research had supported in the past. Previous research had shown evidence for hypothesis one, however it was rejected in this study and results showed that women did not experience more difficulty in finding mentors than men. There were a lot of cross-mentoring relationships found in the study but there was some evidence that showed that women tended to have more women mentors while few men had women as mentors. The majority of mentors were in their mid 40s; however, age had no bearing on the pattern of relationships that emerged between male and female managers. Marital status was found to be a significant factor in the female versus male respondents with the majority of women being unmarried. They had made the decision to postpone marriage at this phase of their career development. Another factor that resulted from the study was that the male respondents tended to have more children than did the women in the survey.

In addition to the demographic variables studied, organizational factors were also analyzed. However, similar to the demographic variables, there was no significant evidence that supported a gender issue. Hypothesis two was rejected because the study did not show that mentoring opportunities for women were negatively influenced by a lack of a formal reward program for mentors, women were found to seek out informal mentoring relationships. Hypotheses three and four were also rejected because no evidence supported intimacy as being a significant issue when it came to mentoring relationships with women. Overall, this study showed no significant differences in mentor access, function, or relationship between genders. Both men and women reported receiving instrumental as well as psychosocial support from their mentors that enhanced their career development.

Implications of the study are very critical because the findings in all of the areas tested refuted previous studies done on this topic. This could mean that there has been an increase in communication available within the workplace and gender differences are becoming less of an issue with equal rights being promoted and supported in most organizations. This study found that mentor roles and functions did not vary between male and female managers and also reinforced the benefits of mentoring and how they can enhance the career development of both parties involved. Findings support the incentives and benefits for the health care industry to implement mentoring programs in their organizations. These programs can promote diversity and provide optimal strategies for managing executive development in the evolving health care industry.

11.3   THE EFFECTS OF ORGANIZATIONAL BEHAVIOR MODIFICATION ON TASK PERFORMANCE

Can managers improve job performance without increasing costs? They may be able to if there is a link between non-financial rewards and increases in task performance. There have been many studies that look at behavioral theory to determine what factors and consequences can be attributed to various behaviors; specifically, improved job performance.

However, there has been no set of factors that can be applied across different types of organizations. This research looks at different types of firms and types of reinforcement and studies the differences.

Alexander D. Stajkovic from the University of California, Irvine, and Fred Luthans from the University of Nebraska (AU: YEAR?), currently study behavior modification and behavioral management, respectively. The researchers tested the effects of the organizational behavior modification (O.B.Mod.) approach on task performance in an organizational setting. O.B.Mod. has roots in operant learning and reinforcement theory.

There were two parts to this study. First, the researchers analyzed a collection of previous studies and developed a summary of past results as a primary meta-analysis for their study. Various criteria were measured for inclusion of a previous study into this analysis, and the effect size for each study was then estimated. The researchers then looked at the homogeneity of effect sizes to test the hypothesis that all samples are drawn from the same population. Any study involving only one subject and any outliers were excluded from further analysis.

After determining the previous studies to be used in the analysis, the researchers came up with four hypotheses. The first hypothesis states that the effect magnitude of O.B.Mod. in service organizations will be lower than in manufacturing organizations. The remaining hypotheses deal with different types of reinforcement. Several re-inforcers of behavior are considered: financial/monetary, non-financial, social, and various combinations. These hypotheses state that

1. each type of reinforcement will produce significant average effects on task performance in manufacturing and service firms,
2. different reinforcement interventions will produce different effects, and
3. each type of reinforcement will produce significant within-class homogeneity of average effects in manufacturing and service organizations.

Next, the researchers used Hedges and Olkin's (1985) meta-analytic method to test each hypothesis.

The results show that there are differences between manufacturing and service organizations when applying the O.B.Mod. approach to improving task performance. This supports Hypothesis 1. The results also show that financial, non-financial, social, and combinations of reinforcements have a significant effect on task performance in manufacturing organizations and in service organizations. In addition, the findings show that different reinforcements lead to different results in both manufacturing and service organizations. These results support the remaining hypotheses.

Although various combinations of reinforcements were shown to have a different relationship with task performance, none of the reinforcements studied were shown to have a significantly stronger effect than others in manufacturing organizations. In service organizations, financial reinforcement produced the strongest effect; however, when financial reinforcement was used in combination with other non-financial reinforcements, the financial reinforcements may contribute to a weaker effect compared to a combination of non-financial reinforcements alone.

For managers, this study shows that there are ways to improve job performance without increasing costs in both manufacturing and service organizations. Non-financial incentives produce essentially the same results as financial incentives. Combinations of non-financial incentives have been shown to improve performance in service organizations; however, the use of reinforcements to improve job performance is stronger in manufacturing organizations. Managers can use the results of this study as a guideline to improve performance without having to increase financial rewards.

11.4   HUMOR AS A MODERATOR OF LEADERSHIP STYLE

Humor as associated with leadership styles is often a topic of discussion. A sense of humor of management leads to higher levels of employee commitment, cohesiveness and performance. Little research has been done to study the connections between the use of humor and management or leadership style. What is currently known about the effects of humor is that of all communicating methods humor is the most effective but also the least understood.

Researchers Bruce J. Avolio of the State University of New York at Binghamton, Jane M. Howell of the University of Western Ontario, and John J. Sosik of Pennsylvania State University (1999) conducted an exploratory study examining how the use of humor moderates a range of leadership styles, including transformational, contingent reward, and laissez-faire leadership. They also examined the use of humor directly related to performance. Previous research led these researchers to predict that the use of humor would have a direct and positive impact on performance.

The researchers distributed surveys to all of the subordinates of each manager who agreed to participate. The sample consisted of 115 leaders representing the top four levels of management and 322 respective subordinates. The leaders were 97 percent male between the age of 29 and 64 years of age. The subordinates were asked to rate the frequency of how often their managers used different leadership behaviors and humor. Eighty-nine percent of the subordinates responded and the results were rated on the basis of one-way analysis of variance and Bartlett tests for homogeneity.

The leadership behavior was surveyed by use of the multifactor leadership questionnaire. The variables measured transformational leadership, contingent reward leadership and laissez-faire leadership. They responded on how often their manager utilized each style. Humor was measured by using information from literature and applied and measured by the frequency of occurrence. The items tested included "uses humor to take the edge off during stressful periods," "uses a funny story to turn an argument in his or her favor," "makes us laugh at ourselves when we are too serious," "uses amusing stories to defuse conflicts," and "uses wit to make friends of the opposition." The company hosting the study provided two additional performance measures. First, the consolidated unit performance represented by the degree to which a manager achieved targeted goals for the year calculated in terms of the percentage of goals met. Secondly, the individual performance appraisal measures representing the manager's overall performance. Control links were used between transformational, contingent reward, and laissez-faire leadership and humor.

The results indicate that transformational leadership was significantly and positively related to the use of humor and to individual and unit performance. Contingent reward leadership was significantly and positively related to the use of humor, but it was negatively related to individual and unit performance. Laissez-faire leadership was significantly and negatively related to the use of humor and to individual and unit performance. The manager's performance appraisal was significantly and positively associated with unit performance in an unmoderated model and in both the low and high humor subsamples.

The research seems to indicate that the use of humor for some leadership behaviors will reduce the negative effects of the chosen leadership style. Such as the positive effects of humor minimizes the effects of the avoidance behaviors displayed by laissez-faire leadership. The researchers could not determine why the moderating effects of humor differed for individual and unit performance. It appears humor creates a climate that allows subordinates to feel better about the unit despite their dissatisfaction with a chosen leadership style.

The implications of the study are determined by each organization's commitment to effective leadership. An organization could utilize this study to train leaders to try humor in situations that could get out of hand. The manager could create the type of relationships among each individual and among units by effectively implementing humor in the work place. They could also vary the styles of leadership along with humor to have a stronger impact on the performance of their subordinates. If managers used the information provided in this research, the impact would be direct and specific. They could gauge the different types of leadership behaviors with different types of humor and predetermine the effectiveness based on the composition of the group.

11.5   EFFECTS OF GENDER ON LEADER EMERGENCE

There has been a considerable amount of research done on the sex and gender role on leader emergence. It has been consistently shown that men more often emerge as leaders than women. However, recent evidence suggests that the female role in society has changed, and some of the barriers that prevented women from being leaders have gone down. With this big change on female roles in society, what are the effects of sex and gender roles on leader emergence now? The researchers Kent and Moss (1994) decided to empirically test the effects of gender role on leader emergence.

The participants were 122 undergraduate, mostly non-working, business students enrolled in one of three upper-division courses in business policy or organizational behavior at a large Southeastern university. Seven students were eliminated from the study because they did not fully complete all necessary requirements, reducing the final participants to 115, with 67 men and 48 women. All agreed to complete questionnaires at the end of the semester.

Group members worked together on several required case presentations or written case analyses, depending on the class throughout the semester. These tasks were considered to be gender-neutral compared to other masculine tasks like repairing machinery or feminine tasks like planning a wedding budget. Doing the assignments required the students to have a great amount of interaction outside of class. With the great amount of interaction with each other, it provided the opportunity to develop relatively strong perceptions about their group leader's behaviors as well as their own.

By comparing individuals' scores on the Bern Sex-Role Inventory (BSRI) to the medians for the entire study group on masculinity and femininity, each individual was assigned one of the four gender role categories, masculine, androgynous, feminine, and undifferentiated.

Leaders emergence was assessed using a three-item scale they developed in previous research. These items suggested that the emergent leaders in groups talk more, participate more actively, and make more attempts to influence the group. The following questions were used for measures: Please rate the extent to which you and each member of your group

1.   assumed a leadership role,
2.   led the conversation, and
3.   influenced group goals and decisions (1 for never and 7 for always).

The three-item measure allowed the possibility of more than one leader by not forcing subjects to choose between two or more group members who each played significant roles in leading the group.

The results revealed that masculinity was definitely correlated with self-perceived leader emergence and group-perceived leader emergence. Almost the same number of men and women were categorized as being androgynous. The most significant finding in this study is that masculinity is still an important predictor of the emergence of leadership. Secondly, when the percentage of women in a group is controlled, the women are slightly more likely to emerge as leaders than men are. Thirdly, it was found that gender role is a better predictor of leadership emergence than sex. Lastly, by comparing gender role on the self and group perceptions made clear that those that are categorized as masculine and androgynous were not only perceived by their group as leaders, but by themselves as well, unlike those categorized as feminine and undifferentiated.

The findings of this study suggests that androgynous individuals and women are not only more likely to emerge as leaders in school settings, but this idea will drift into the business setting as well. This implies that people are more accepting than before of women being in control and that the traditional gender role is weakening.

11.6   TRUST AND DISTRUST IN ORGANIZATIONS

Trust and distrust have always been viewed as inversely correlated to each other. In this paper, the researchers aim to disprove theories on trust and distrust that have spanned more than 40 years. They propose a new framework for understanding simultaneous trust and distrust within relationships, grounded in assumptions of multidimensionality and the inherent tensions of relationships.

Researchers Roy J. Lewicki of Ohio State University, Daniel J. McAllister, and Robert J. Bies, both of Georgetown University (1998) propose new definitions of trust and distrust and relate them to each other in different ways from what has been done in the past. They argue that trust and distrust are separate but linked dimensions.

The researchers point out two core differences in their study. The first is that relationships are multifaceted or multiplex. This enables groups to hold different views of each other at the same time. The second is that balance and consistency in one's cognitions and perceptions are more likely to be temporary and transitional states. Simple and fast solutions are not always the end result of the tensions created by the states of imbalance and inconsistency that people are more likely to be in.

What the researchers found was that trust and distrust were not reciprocal of each other. Low distrust did not necessarily mean high trust and the same went for high distrust did not translate to low trust. These four sub-dimensions of trust and distrust each have different characteristics that make them unique. That is why they are not perfectly correlated to one another. This thesis is also very dependent on the fact that ambivalence with respect to trust and distrust are very possible. It is also important to point out that with all of this evidence it is still possible for trust and distrust to coexist.

The researchers believe that even though more trust has been viewed as beneficial while distrust is detrimental to organizations, the potential for productive distrust may contribute to, rather than, detract from, economic order and efficiency.

The implications of this study point to a need for individuals in organizations to trust their fellow staff members, but at the same time ensure that proper monitoring is in place of what all employees are doing. A classic example is the need for control systems in organizations. These systems are able to function in a culture of trust.

11.7 WORK-RELATED DISTRESS RESULTING FROM CONTACT WITH AIDS PATIENTS

The researchers hypothesized that a nurse's exposure to AIDS patients as part of her job is positively associated with distress (negative mood) at work. If this is true the researchers sought to identify factors which may reduce the negative effects of caring for AIDS patients. They predicted that both organizational and social support would moderate the relationship between the extent of exposure and the negative mood.

Researchers Jennifer M. George, Thomas F. Reed, Karen A. Ballard, Jessie Colin, and Jane Fielding (1993) sent out questionnaires to 1,600 nurses who were members of the New York State Nurses Association. A random sample of nurses in New York City, Buffalo, Rochester, Syracuse, and Albany were sent 800 of the questionnaires because these cities would have the highest concentration of AIDS patients. The remaining 800 questionnaires were randomly sent to the remaining nurses from the association. 256 completed surveys were returned, a 16 percent response rate.

The researchers collected data on five measures including: negative and positive moods, extent of exposure, organizational support, social support, and negative affectivity. They measured mood by using a Job Affect Scale and summing the responses to six negative mood items and six positive mood items to arrive at negative and positive mood scores. The researchers used a three-item scale to determine the perceived extent of a nurse's exposure to AIDS patients. They used a Survey of Perceived Organizational Support and a Social Support Questionnaire to measure the amounts of perceived organizational and social support the nurses were getting. Finally they measured negative affectivity as a control variable. Negative affectivity is a personality trait predisposing an individual to experience negative affectivity, be dissatisfied, have negative views of self and others, and interpret ambiguous stimuli negatively. They used a 14-item questionnaire to measure this trait.

Before the survey was taken and the results were tabulated and interpreted the researchers had formulated three distinct hypotheses. They are listed below:

1. The extent of a nurse's exposure to the AIDS patients as part of the nursing role is positively associated with negative mood at work.
2. Organizational support moderates the relationship between extent of exposure to AIDS patients and negative mood at work; the relationship is strongest when organizational support is low and weakest when organizational support is high.
3. Social support moderates the relationship between extent of exposure to AIDS patients and negative mood at work; the relationship is strongest when social support is unsatisfactory and weakest when social support is satisfactory.

In essence the researchers believed that there was a positive relationship between having negative moods at work and a nurse's perceived contact and exposure to AIDS patients. This negative mood could be tempered by organizations providing support to their nurses including counseling, time off, and reassignment. Organizational support will also give nurses a better understanding about the virus and their risk of infection based upon the work they perform. In addition the researchers felt that social support was another factor which would help moderate a nurse's negative mood brought on by exposure to AIDS patients. The researchers felt that the social support would give nurses positive self-esteem and the ability to talk to others as a coping mechanism.

The researchers tabulated the data and ran the necessary regressions in order to formulate conclusions about their hypotheses. In general the data supported the researchers hypotheses. The data showed that there was indeed a correlation between exposure and negative mood. The data also allowed the researchers to conclude that when organizational support and social support were high, the relationship between exposure to AIDS and negative mood was weakest. When support was low the relationship between exposure to AIDS patients and negative mood was strongest. The researchers did this while controlling the possibility that people with negative personality traits might skew the data.

This research has important implications for nurses in the field and health care organizations. The data suggest that health care organizations need to provide adequate support to nurses that deal with AIDS patients and that they should monitor their psychological well being. Additional research may be done to determine what are the most effective means of providing the support that nurses need from both a social and organizational standpoint.

REFERENCES

Avolio, B. J., Howell, J. M., & Sosik, J. J. (1999). A funny thing happened on the way to the bottom line: Humor as a moderator of the leadership style effects. *Academy of Management Journal, 42*(2), 219-227.

Fox, M. L., Dwyer, D. J., & Ganster, D. C. (1993). Effects of stressful job demands and job control on physiological and attitudinal outcomes in a hospital setting. *Academy of Management Journal, 36*(2), 289-318.

George, J. M., Reed, T. F., Ballard, K. A., Colin, J., & Fielding, J. (1993). Contact with AIDS patients as a source of work-related distress: Effects of organizational and social support. *Academy of Management Journal, 36*(1), 151-171.

Kent, R. L., & Moss, S. E. (1994). Effects of sex and gender role on leader emergence. *Academy of Management Journal, 37*(5), 1335-1346.

Lewicki, R. J., McAllister, D. M., & Bies, R. J. (1998). Trust and distrust: New relationships and realities. *Academy of Management Review, 23*(3), 438-458.

Stajkovic, A. D., & Luthans, F. (1997) A meta-analysis of the effects of organizational behavior modification on task performance. *Academy of Management Journal, 40*(5), 1122-1150.

Walsh, A. M., & Borkowski, S. C. (1999). Cross-gender career development in the health care industry. *Health Care Management Review, 24*(3), 7-22.

CHAPTER 12

INSTITUTIONAL ISSUES IN HEALTH SYSTEMS

This chapter addresses a number of organizational and institutional issues in health delivery services.

The first study's focus is on managing hospitals in turbulent times. It attempts to discover what organizational changes contribute to the closing of hospitals. The organizational changes evaluated were two core changes consisting of ownership changes and major service changes, and five peripheral changes consisting of multi-hospital system affiliation, corporate restructuring, addition of long-term care unit, down sizing and chief executive officer (CEO) succession. Control variables such as hospital size, hospital age, ownership, etc. were also included in the statistical model. The results indicated that ownership change was the core structure that affected hospital closure. Corporate restructuring, downsizing and CEO succession were the peripheral changes that affected hospital closure. Organizational changes should generally not be used to avoid hospital closure.

The second study shows that there is a need for communication in the process of developing corporate mission statements. The approach taken was a case study in one firm. A total of 152 members of management in the same firm were asked to evaluate six mission statements developed by nine

Proven Solutions for Improving Health and Lowering Health Care Costs, pages 169–183.
Copyright © 2003 by Information Age Publishing, Inc.
All rights of reproduction in any form reserved.
ISBN: 1-59311-000-6 (paper), 1-59311-001-4 (cloth)

top management members. The study showed that both management level and department affiliation affected the ranking of such issues as customer satisfaction and quality of work life. The study points out the need to devote considerable effort and to ensure wide participation in the development of a corporate mission statement. And following its development extensive communication and wide dissemination of the mission statement is necessary for its acceptance.

The third study explores how collaborative know-how can be learned by organizations that collaborate with other organizations with arrangements such as joint ventures, consortia, contractual agreements and informal cooperation. The study showed that organizations learn from collaborative ventures by developing skills in identifying potential collaborators, negotiating the form and specifics of agreements, managing and monitoring the arrangements, knowing when to terminate them, and transferring knowledge. Collaborative experience must be linked with internalization of the lessons learned and assimilation into know-how that can be used by the organization in future situations.

The fourth study describes the network effectiveness of four community mental health systems. The study was performed in four U.S. cities consisting of Tucson, Arizona; Albuquerque, New Mexico; Providence, Rhode Island; and Akron, Ohio. From the study of the four cities, the researchers concluded that all forms of network integration are not alike and are likely to have different consequences for overall network effectiveness. Networks integrated and coordinated centrally, through a single core agency, are likely to be more effective than dense, cohesive networks integrated in a decentralized way.

The fifth study explored interorganizational links and innovation in hospital services. The researchers conducted a longitudinal study of over 400 California hospitals over a ten-year period in order to examine the relationship between interorganizational links and innovation. The focus was on service innovations within each hospital. The results showed that innovation was significantly more likely among hospitals that had structural, institutional or resource links. However, administrative links and market concentration were negatively related to innovation. Hospital size was positively related to innovation. The general conclusion was that interorganizational links are efficient mechanisms for exchanges of technological capabilities and knowledge.

The sixth study explored the effects of leadership style and cultural orientation on the performance of group and individual tasks. The two types of leadership studied were transactional and transformational. And the two types of cultural orientation were individualistic and collectivistic. The results showed that transactional leaders inspired a higher quality aspiration in Caucasians. Asians working with a transformational leader outperformed those working with a transactional leader. In general, the study revealed that the same leadership style can be perceived differently and can have different effects on motivation and performance for followers from different cultural groups.

The seventh study explored the benefits of reciprocity in negotiations. The research environments were role play negotiations between 25 MBA students and 25 former MBA students, generally employed at the time of the study. The results of the study showed that communications of all types were reciprocated more often than would typically be predicted. The implications of the study can be viewed as the need for managers to be able to constructively solve conflict, especially in an inter-corporation dispute.

The eighth and final study covers organizational responsiveness to work-family issues. The data base of the study consists of 175 responses of human resource executives from a wide variety of corporations in the United States. Work-family areas explored cover leave programs, flexible work options, dependent care programs, financial benefits, miscellaneous supportive benefits and overall work-family responsiveness. The results show that companies which perform exit interviews and employee surveys show the most responsiveness to work-family related issues. Also managers of companies that offered good support packages related to work-family issues felt that the productivity of their employees was higher.

A variety of organizational and institutional issues were covered in this chapter. Managers can benefit from studying the results reported by researchers of the various studies.

12.1 MANAGING HOSPITALS DURING INDUSTRY RESTRUCTURING

How do organizational changes affect hospital survival? Do core and peripheral changes affect hospital survival differently? How do simultaneous organizational changes affect hospital survival? Dramatic environmental changes in the economic and institutional environment of hospitals have caused increases in hospital closings and mass organizational changes. Strategies that used to be used only in the corporate sector, such as downsizing, diversification, and alliances are some of the trends now seen in the health care sector.

Data was collected from community hospitals (nonfederal short-term facilities whose services are available to the public) in the continental United States over the period from 1981 through 1994. Data for the study was obtained from three sources: the American Hospital Association (AHA) Annual Survey of Hospitals, the Area Resource File, and the AHA Hospital Guides, Part B: Multi-hospital Systems. Hospitals remained in the study until they were closed or right censored (the closure event had not occurred and the hospital remained open or the occurrence of the closure was uncertain). The data set consisted of 66,909 repeated observations of hospitals or hospital-year observations.

The study by Lee and Alexander (1999) tested four hypotheses consisting of:

1. Core organizational changes will increase the rate of hospital closure,
2. Peripheral organizational change will reduce the rate of hospital closure,
3. Simultaneous core changes will increase the rate of hospital closure, and
4. Simultaneous peripheral changes will increase the rate of hospital closure. These hypotheses were tested by a series of regression models.

The dependent variable was hospital closure. The independent variables were changes in a hospital's core and peripheral structures. Two core changes were examined: ownership changes and major service changes. Five peripheral changes were examined: multi-hospital system affiliation, corporate restructuring, addition of a long-term care unit, downsizing, and chief executive officer (CEO) succession.

Organizational control variables such as age, size, ownership, occupancy, operational efficiency, teaching status, rural location, and institutional ties with accrediting organizations, national associations, and insurance groups were incorporated into the study. An additional variable, Missing, was used to indicate cases with missing values on the organizational change variables in order to retain a complete set of observations. Four environmental control variables were incorporated into the study that were assessed on the following three levels: the level of resources available in the local market, the level of competition in the local market, and the level of market uncertainty.

Most changes occurred in the hospital's peripheral structure rather than in the core structure. Ownership change was the only core change that was significantly associated with hospital closure. Corporate restructuring, downsizing, and CEO succession were the peripheral changes that were significantly associated with hospital closure. Other than specialty change, adding organizational and environmental variables reduced the effects of individual organizational changes on hospital closure. Hospital characteristics and environmental conditions seem more important in explaining hospital closure than do organizational changes.

The study calls into doubt the general belief that organizational changes improve the survival chances of hospitals. Most organizational changes had either no impact on hospital survival or adversely affected community hospital survival. Organizational changes can, at times, place hospitals at greater risk. Many organizational changes showed positive relationships with hospital closure. Although specialty change had a negative effect on hospital closure, possibly because this change is more strategic in nature and may have been more carefully planned and implemented. Multiple core changes showed a negative relationship with hospital closure while multiple peripheral changes had a more positive relationship with closure. More research is needed to examine the issue of organizational capability in implementing change.

What then is a hospital left to do if organizational changes are not beneficial on an overall basis? Hospital leaders should be cautious to implement mass changes to the core organization and need to carefully consider how proposed changes will affect the operation of the hospital. Given the constant turbulence in the industry, hospitals must focus on strategy and anticipate changes in the environment in order to survive.

12.2   THE NEED FOR COMMUNICATION OF CORPORATE MISSION STATEMENTS

The researchers of this study deal with the issue of corporate mission and how its priorities change between the different levels of management. This is a problem, as it is widely felt that corporate success relies heavily on the ability to internalize the corporate mission. Reports have shown in the past that the mission of a company never gets communicated to the employees who carry out the everyday jobs, but rather gets posted on the walls of the senior management office suites.

The study was conducted by Harvey Brightman from Georgia State University, and Lutfus Sayeed from West Virginia University (1994). The sample for the study consisted of a vice president and a 152 member management team from a large technological firm. This particular division of the firm consisted of four line and four staff departments with six managerial levels. The staff departments were represented by accounting, human resources, marketing, and operations, while the line departments provided the technical resources to the different districts within the division. The 153 person sample, consisted of a vice president (VP), 8 department managers, and 144 professional employees.

The researchers felt that the optimal time to conduct a study on the congruence of a mission statement, is when the company is going through a transition. This particular firm had appointed a vice president only nine months earlier thus making the firm a good candidate for the study.

The division's mission statement was developed by the vice president and the eight department managers and when finalized, six distinct mission statements resulted. The six mission statements covered customer satisfaction, performance standards, teamwork, quality of work life, contextual leadership, and accountability.

Brightman and Sayeed's goal was to test the extent of the communication of the mission statements, and to determine whether the organizational level had an effect on the priority given to the different statements. They were able to do this by studying the congruence of the priorities between the management levels and the vice president.

A questionnaire was given to each of the participants that contained 15 forced pair comparisons between the six different mission statements. The mission importance score was calculated by the number of times that a particular mission was chosen over the other five mission statements.

The theory behind this study began with research conducted by other researchers, which showed that mission statements often include eight components: philosophy, self concept, public image, location, technology, concern for survival, customer service, and product service. The belief is that due to the many distinct components of the mission statements, there is a lack of congruence of mission priorities between the different levels of the organization.

The study found that although the vice president and the management team agreed on the relative ranking of the six mission statements, there were some statistically significant differences. The management team assigned lower importance scores (than the VP) in regards to teamwork and performance standards, while assigning higher scores in the areas of quality of work life and accountability.

The study also showed that both management level and departmental affiliation affected the ranking of customer satisfaction and the quality of work life. On the other hand the analysis revealed that management level alone affected the ranking of the teamwork mission statement.

The main implication of this study is that it brings to light the many distinct aspects of a corporate mission statement, and that if left to their own devices different management levels and departments will focus on what they feel is important. This lack of a clearly communicated mission or strategy can become a major inhibitor to the success of a firm. The need to fully communicate the mission statement and the ranking of the important issues is a more important step than the actual writing of the mission statement itself.

12.3   COLLABORATIVE KNOW-HOW AND THE LEARNING ORGANIZATION

It was found that for firms to learn from their strategic alliances they must internalize their experiences and collaborative know-how must be developed, in order for a firm to benefit in future collaborations. Collaborations include joint-ventures, consortia, equity participation, contractual agreements, and informal cooperation. Companies can develop specialized knowledge via experience and use this knowledge to obtain further bene-fit. Firms that were found to have higher levels of collaborative know-how were found to achieve higher levels of tangible and intangible benefits from their collaborations.

Bernard L. Simonin (1997) of the University of Washington used a large cross sectional sample of companies that can and do compete, and ana-lyzed their effectiveness in learning from collaboration. He sought out to study whether firms learn from the success and failure of collaborations and if they applied these lessons to future collaboration. He found that a firm's experience must be transformed into know-how before it can improve performance. Benefits were divided into tangible benefits inclu-sive of strategic and financial such as generating additional profits, improv-ing market share, and sustaining competitive advantage, and intangible benefits of learning and knowledge such as learning specific skills and competencies, inter-firm cooperation, and learning how to form collabora-tions.

Professor Simonin sent a questionnaire to key executives of large US corporations with experience in domestic and overseas collaboration, that were involved in collaborative efforts for their companies. 192 companies participated and 151 questionnaires were fully completed and utilized. The strategic alliances that were still active and used in the study had an average life of 6 years.

A significant result from this study is the proof that firms do learn from collaborations by developing skills in identifying potential collaborators, negotiating the form and specifics of collaborative agreements, managing and monitoring the arrangements, knowing when to terminate them, and transferring knowledge. It was also found that these benefits are not attain-able by experience alone. Experience must be linked with internalization of the lessons learned and assimilation into know-how that can be used by the firm in future situations. This point is critical to gain benefit from col-laboration and is consistent with building a learning organization.

Limitations of this study include error due to single respondents to the questionnaires. Only one executive from each company was used to supply data for analysis. This may have resulted in skewed biased information. In the future, further testing could be performed using both subjective and objective information on collaborations within multiple companies. This information should be from multiple sources.

12.4   NETWORK EFFECTIVENESS OF FOUR COMMUNITY MENTAL HEALTH SYSTEMS

In the mental health industry the relation between one part of an organiza-tion with another part of the same organization has been a major concern for quite some time. But recently networking outside of the organization has taken on a greater importance with the success of the organization. These changes have been attributed to for-profit firms, but organizations in not-for-profit and public sectors are also increasingly turning to various forms of cooperative alliances as a way of enhancing competitiveness and effectiveness that would not be possible through the traditional governance mechanisms of market or hierarchy. In the area of community-based health care and social services for such groups as the homeless, people with severe mental illness, drug and alcohol abusers, and the elderly, a focus on organizational issues in one agency is not sufficient, since this only provides how one provider is performing their one particular specialty out of the many services described above. If the overall well-being of the clients is the goal, then the network as a whole must be judged. This is due to the integrated and coordinated actions of many different agencies that provide shelter, transportation, food, and other various support services.

Researchers Keith Provan and H. Brinton Milward (1995) published a paper testing the results of networking effectiveness in four U.S. cities: Tucson, Arizona; Albuquerque, New Mexico; Providence, Rhode Island; and Akron, Ohio. These cities were chosen on the basis that they were large enough to contain the full criteria needed to demonstrate network effectiveness between organizations, but not large enough so that the data collected was too large to handle. All four cities also had one major mental health agency whose role was to coordinate the services of other community agencies. Finally, two cities were selected from states with high levels of per capita health spending (New Mexico and Arizona). With this in place, the researchers proceeded to collect data that would demonstrate how network effectiveness is essential to the overall success of organizations in health services.

The quantitative and qualitative data collected at each of these four cities could be categorized in three different categories:
1. individual level,

2. organizational/network level, and
3. network level.

At the individual level, data was collected from a 5 percent random sample of adult clients in each of these cities who depended on agencies for continued treatment. These adults were not institutionalized so the study would emphasize how networking was essential to helping out these clients. Data was also collected from the clients' families and their case managers to get a multi-perspective approach. All results were analyzed to see if there were similarities and differences between the cities and the groups.

From an organizational/network level, the focus of the study was how the separate organizations were linked among each other to make up the network. This data was broken down into two categories: density and centralization. To measure density, key personnel at each agency were asked to indicate if their agency was involved with every other agency listed on the survey in five different types of service links: referrals sent, referrals received, case coordination, joint programs, and service contracts. The personnel were asked to report only cases in which mentally ill patients were involved, not just interaction as a whole. This was important in establishing network effectiveness in the mental health industry, not just the industry as a whole. To measure centralization, the service and organizational density scores for the core agency were taken out of the density scores mentioned above and the figures were re-computed and differences noted. This was done to see if integration and coordination of services across the network would be enhanced when the decisions related to mental health clients was concentrated in a single organization.

From a network level, funding from outside sources may play a major role in external control of an organization. Data collected in this area had to do with the original selection of the four cities in the area of level per capita mental health spending. This data was important in demonstrating how external control and resource munificence was important in the researcher's theory of network effectiveness.

The results of the research in the four cities can be broken down into many categories. In the area of client/families, the network in Providence was considered to be the most effective in meeting clients' needs, followed by Albuquerque, Tucson, and Akron. The managers/therapists felt that the network in Albuquerque was the best, followed by Tucson, Providence, and Akron. In the area of density and centrality, Providence had the highest core-agency linkage score, but the lowest level of linkages (density), which would indicate a highly centralized control system. The managers/therapists felt that this highly centralized system took away their power, and graded them lower accordingly. Akron was next, followed by Albuquerque, and then Tucson, which exhibited characteristics of a highly decentralized but integrated system (high density). This finding is important because Providence had the best score in the area of client/families, which would indicate that a highly centralized control system helps the network as a whole. Another important finding was that Providence had the advantage of high state funding, (external control, high resource munificence) as well as a highly stable system that had been in place for more than 20 years. Conversely, Tucson and Akron were both relatively new systems, while Albuquerque was a relatively stable system, although it had poor funding and poor integration across the system.

From the study of the four cities, the researchers concluded that all forms of network integration are not alike and are likely to have different consequences for overall network effectiveness. Networks integrated and coordinated centrally, through a single core agency, are likely to be more effective than dense, cohesive networks integrated in a decentralized way.

The implications of this study in the business world would demonstrate that differences in network effectiveness could be explained in the areas of centralized integration, external control, stability, and resource munificence. Instead of just focusing on one perspective, multiple perspectives allow a greater in-depth analysis of interorganizational relations and networks. The researchers believe that a combination of network structure and network context is important in developing good network effectiveness. In the area of network structure, centralized integration and direct non-fragmented external control play major factors in establishing good network effectiveness. In the area of network context, system stability, and high resource munificence contribute to good network effectiveness.

12.5 ALLIANCES AND INNOVATION IN HOSPITAL SERVICES

Interorganizational links have been studied extensively in recent literature. They have shown benefit to organizations through increased efficiency, stability, and legitimacy, among other factors, but no one theory of interorganizational links is salient. At the same time, due to increasing dispersion of technical competence and increasing complexity and uncertainty, innovation has become increasingly difficult for individual firms. This study aims to fill two important gaps in the literature: (1) examining interorganizational links as well as a way of modeling and understanding organizational conduct as it relates to firm-level innovation, and (2) by conducting a longitudinal study.

Researchers James Goes from the University of Alaska Southeast, and Seung Ho Park from Rutgers University (1997), conducted a longitudinal study of over 400 California hospitals over ten years to examine the relationship between interorganizational links and innovation. The study focused on hospitals as the unit of analysis and concentrated specifically on service innovations. The authors conceptualized several ways in which interorganizational links may influence innovation, and tested their theories based on the resource dependence model and open-systems perspective.

The main theoretical underpinning of the study is based on the resource dependence model and suggests that organizations are dependent on their task environment, and exchange and reciprocity are essential for success in managing resources (and thus achieving competitive advantage). The authors categorized interorganizational links as structural, administrative, institutional, and resource links, and derived hypotheses for their effects on innovation adoption in each category. All of the hypotheses suggested a positive relationship between the independent variable (type of link) and the dependent variable (likeliness of adopting service innovation).

The authors justified the choice of hospitals as the unit of analysis because the health care industry has exhibited increasing technical complexity and environmental turbulence, and thus has established strong interorganizational ties. Data collection mainly used archival data available from State agencies, but also incorporated interviews, field observations, mailed surveys and other data. Innovation was measured based on an inventory of 135 separate service offerings reported to the State.

Structural links were measured as an indication of whether the hospitals were part of a multihospital system. Administrative links measured the extent to which hospitals contracted for management services with another hospital. Institutional links were measured as the hospitals' involvement in institutional or trade organizations. Resource links were measured as the total dollar value of major transactions between a hospital and a related hospital (shared ownership). Statistical analyses including time-series multiple regression was applied to evaluate the influence of the predictor variables on innovation adoption. Control variables included urbanization, affluence, market concentration, size, and ownership.

The results of the study supported the authors' hypotheses that innovation was significantly more likely among hospitals that had structural, institutional, or resource links. Interestingly however, the results showed that administrative links were significantly negatively related to innovation. Affluence was found to have no significant effect, market concentration had an inverse effect, and size was directly related. Privately owned hospitals were less likely to innovate than not-for-profit hospitals, and no significant difference was found between public and not-for-profit hospitals with respect to innovation. Generally speaking, the results suggest that interorganizational links are efficient mechanisms for exchanges of technological capabilities and knowledge.

The results of this study are significant for managers and business analysts in understanding and responding to environmental trends and competitive strategies. The significant relationship between interorganizational links and service innovation suggest that the links are a strong predictor of innovation and may serve to reduce resource dependency and thus increase competitive advantage.

12.6 LEADERSHIP STYLE AND CULTURAL ORIENTATION

With the growing diversity in America's workforce, today's leaders need to recognize that different styles of leadership will have varying degrees of success depending on the followers' cultural orientations. The problem that the researchers set out to address was determining what sort of leadership (Transactional or Transformational) is good for what cultural orientation (Individualistic or Collectivistic) of the followers.

Researchers Dong J. Jung of San Diego State University, and Bruce J. Avolio of the State University of New York at Birmingham (1999), conducted a study of 347 students (153 Asians and 194 Caucasians) of business at the School of Management of a large public university in the Northeastern United States. In their research, they manipulated transformational and transactional leadership styles and compared them in individual and group task conditions to determine whether they had different impacts on individualists and collectivists performing a brainstorming task.

Their study used a completely crossed two-by-two experimental design that manipulated leadership style and task structure with Caucasian and Asian samples. Groups from each cultural background were instructed to behave in either an individual setting or as part of a larger group to solve a problem. Different segments of these groups received instructions from a leader scripted to perform in either a transactional or transformational manner.

After the prescribed task was completed, the groups' results were tallied and compared to their survey results that incorporated seventeen items adapted from a leadership questionnaire.

The results of the study were interesting in that they did not exactly match up with the researchers' expectations. Transactional leaders inspired the generation of more ideas in Caucasians, but transformational leaders evoked the generation of ideas with a long-term orientation. Meanwhile, Asians working with a transformational leader outperformed those working with a transactional leader, but transformational leadership did not have a significant impact on the generation of long-term ideas.

The study revealed that the same leadership style can be perceived differently and can have different effects on motivation and performance for followers from different cultural groups. And a group versus individual psychological orientation may or may not be the same as a cultural orientation. The implications for managers are that there is a greater need for diversity training now that we are seeing a wider cultural representation in the workforce. Different leadership styles will garner different results under homogeneous circumstances, but cultural variables add a complexity heretofore unseen.

12.7   RECIPROCITY IN NEGOTIATIONS

Conflicts within and between organizations are common, often costing time and money. Such conflicts are especially noticeable in new organizational structures, where such new structures release conflicts that the old structures contained with rules and specific hierarchies. The key to reducing these conflicts is to understand how conflict spirals start and how to break them before they damage the organization.

Researchers Jeanne M. Brett of Northwestern University, Debra L. Shapiro of the University of North Carolina at Chapel Hill, and Anne L. Lytle of the Hong Kong University of Science and Technology (1996), tested four hypotheses concerning the effectiveness of three strategies for breaking conflict spirals. This was done by observing an extensive role-play dispute set in the business environment using 25 MBA students who were currently enrolled in a conflict negotiations class and 25 "outsiders" who were working or were former MBA students.

Participants were assigned the role of chief executive officer (CEO) of two printing companies which were competitors. There were 14 dyads in which the outsiders were representatives of Rapid Printing and 11 dyads of students representing Scott Computers. Each dyad tape recorded its 60 minutes of conflict negotiations. Eleven students who were not involved in the negotiations were asked to code the statements made in each negotiation using an accepted coding scheme.

The results of this study showed that communications of all types were reciprocated more often than would typically be predicted, proving the hypothesis that reciprocation occurs. It also confirmed that reciprocation of contentious communications was not limited to negotiations playing one role of the other or having insider status. (A reciprocated contentious communication was said to have occurred each time a negotiator used a rights or power communication and the other negotiator responded with a rights or power communication.)

The implications of the results of this study for business are critical, especially in a day and age when there are many joint ventures, mergers, acquisitions, and networks. Managers need to be able to constructively solve conflict, especially in an inter-corporation dispute. Given that conflict in and between people and organizations is likely to increase with increased reliance on teams and the necessity of contacts between people and firms with different cultures and values, the results of this study have both practical and theoretical implications.

12.8 RESPONSIVENESS TO WORK-FAMILY ISSUES AND MANAGERIAL ORIENTATION

The question of what makes one organization more responsive to work-family issues while others are not is the focus of this paper from the *Academy of Management Journal*. The issues under scrutiny in this paper include flexible work options, job sharing, and dependent care services. With the influx of women in the workforce over the past 5 years, this paper is questioning whether businesses are adopting policies to help employees manage their work and personal lives.

The researchers, Milliken, Martins, and Morgan (1998), sent letters to a random sample of 1,000 human resource executives at companies around the United States. 175 usable responses accounting for an 18 percent response rate were used to tabulate the results. The research was to determine which factors had an effect on the responsiveness to work family issues. Was it based on the number of female employees in the company or was it based on those companies which hired the most female employees over the past 5 years? Were companies which had higher percentages of women in senior management positions more likely to be responsive to the needs of work family issues? The paper also questioned the use of exit interviews in the openness of a company to implement work-family benefits. Lastly, the survey looked at the effect of the human resource managers' impact on the work-family benefits if the manager believed that satisfaction with work-family benefits were related to productivity.

Work-family responsive items measured in this paper include leave programs, flexible work options, dependent care programs, financial benefits, miscellaneous supportive benefits, and overall work-family responsiveness. The researchers found that institutions with larger numbers of women were not more responsive to the employees' family needs. Even those companies which have recently, over the past 5 years, had an influx of female workers did not have any extra support for family issues. It was discussed that this could be due to the fact that although many more women are entering the work force, many are entering in part-time positions with few if any benefits.

The results indicated that women in top management positions did little to help the cause of work-family responsiveness in their respective organizations. This was hypothesized to be just the opposite case since it was believed that women would be more sympathetic to work-family issues. A suggestion for why this is not so is that women at the top of companies must often work hard to fit in just like the male top managers; therefore, it is in their best interest to refrain from being too supportive of women's issues.

Companies that perform exit interviews and employee surveys actually had the most significant support for a company's responsiveness to work-family related issues. It was ascertained that the companies that conduct surveys and exit interviews often learn what the employees need and were more positive in making sure the employees were happy and productive members of the company. The companies whose human resource manager felt that productivity was higher when employees were happy with the work-family benefits also indicated that they offered good packages to the employees.

The impact of this study on business is especially important for human resource managers and should be looked at by the upper management team members of both genders. If production is higher in companies which take care of their employees with responsiveness to work-family issues then it is beneficial for all managers to take a longer look at how they can best help their employees whether it be through leave programs, flexible work options, dependent care programs, financial benefits, or miscellaneous supportive benefits. In conclusion the research findings support that managers will respond differently to the same constraints dependent on how they perceive the organization they work in.

REFERENCES

Brett, J. M., Shapiro, D. L., & Lytle, A. L. (1996). Breaking the bonds of reciprocity in negotiations. *Academy of Management Journal, 41*(4), 410-424.

Brightman, H. J., & Sayeed, L. (1994). The impact of organizational level and affiliation on corporate mission priorities. *Journal of Education for Business, 69*(January/February), 167-178.

Goes, J. B., & Park, S. H. (1997). Interorganizational links and innovation: The case of hospital services. *The Academy of Management Journal, 40*(3), 673-696.

Jung, D. I., & Avolio, B. J. (1999). Effects of leadership style and followers' cultural orientation on performance in group and individual task conditions. *Academy of Management Journal, 42*(2), 208-218.

Lee, S. D., & Alexander, J. A. (1999). Managing hospitals in turbulent times: Do organizational changes improve hospital survival? *Health Services Research, 34*(4), 923-939.

Milliken, F. J., Martins, L. L., & Morgan, H. (1998). Explaining organizational responsiveness to work-family issues: The role of human resource executives as issue interpreters. *Academy of Management Journal, 41*(5), 580-592.

Provan, K. G., & Milward, H. B. (1995). A preliminary theory of interorganizational network effectiveness: A comparative study of four community hospital health systems. *Administrative Science Quarterly, 40*, 1-33.

Simonin, B. L. (1997). The importance of collaborative know-how: An empirical test of the learning organization. *Academy of Management Journal, 40*(5), 1150-1174.

CHAPTER 13

MANAGERIAL ISSUES IN HEALTH SYSTEMS

This chapter looks at management issues in health care organizations. Areas covered include entrepreneurial failure, organizational learning, decision making by health service managers, and other issues.

The first study addresses professional service organizations and focus. The researchers evaluated advantages and disadvantages of focusing on outpatient surgery centers as the primary example of focus. The major conclusion from the study is that while focusing may cause an organization to lose economies of scope and scale, these losses can sometimes be superseded by other economies such as fewer support staff, less capital investment, and greater market penetration in the focussed segment due to better service.

The second study focuses on an analysis of nursing home outcomes based on the attributes of both the residents and the facilities. The sample consisted of over 4,400 nursing home residents in the state of Massachusetts. Data was collected on patient histories including assistance in daily living (ADL) status. The results show that the more fragile Medicaid patients showed quicker deterioration in ADL functional status than similar patients who show the same demographic and clinical conditions. Also, the more physically impaired patients were at greater risk for increased

Proven Solutions for Improving Health and Lowering Health Care Costs, pages 185–199.
Copyright © 2003 by Information Age Publishing, Inc.
All rights of reproduction in any form reserved.
ISBN: 1-59311-000-6 (paper), 1-59311-001-4 (cloth)

cognitive and behavioral problems. Finally, residents with mental dysfunctions showed a greater decline in comparison with similar patients.

The third study focuses on case management (CM), client risk factors and service use. Chart data was used in a retrospective study of nearly 900 cases from eight geographically dispersed areas, all part of the Alzheimer's Disease Demonstration Project. Although numerous results were produced by this study, the more important one is that effective resource utilization is a key issue for managed care organizations. Through the clarification of CM activities, studies such as this one can be used to improve staffing, treatment protocols and client service outcomes.

The fourth study explores reasoning and entrepreneurial failure. The study describes entrepreneurial initiatives as real options in bundles indicating that there are interrelated effects to evaluate when attempting to describe what leads to the success or failure of the entrepreneurial process. The implications of real options reasoning can provide the conceptual foundation for a new perspective on the dynamics of performance, survival, and choice in entrepreneurship.

The fifth study explores decision making by health service managers. The question posed was: when making decision are managers more likely to optimize or satisfice the requirement? Recent research has shown that to understand a manager's decision making process you must understand the model that they apply to the decision making process. The study is a panel study based on interviews of 16 managers employed by the British health service. The study determined between 9 and 24 factors as those that influence the decision making by the managers. The most common factor, used by 87 percent of the subjects, was "political." Only 30 percent viewed "quality" and "vision" as important. This study confirms that decisions being made by managers are made to satisfy the requirements versus optimizing the resultant outcomes.

The sixth study explores the attitudes and behaviors of integrated physicians. The term, integrated physicians, refers to physicians who function in a system with vertical integration of hospital and community physicians. The survey was principally based on a survey of over 6,800 physicians. The study's focus was on physician autonomy, physician participation in decision making, physician commitment to the hospital, and physician trust to the primary hospital. The results of the study focussed on economic linkage, administrative involvement and admitting behavior. On average, physicians spend 18 percent of their practice time in hospital-based practice and derive 25 percent of their income from salaried employment. Less than 10 percent of physicians were found to occupy board roles and nearly 13 percent performed committee roles. Admission loyalty exerted a positive effect on commitment and trust, and admission volume positively affected commitment. The final conclusion was that economic linkage can improve certain work relationships which promote admitting behavior to the primary hospital.

The seventh and final study explores learners and organizational learning. Although the study has a manufacturing setting it is relevant to health care management. The focus of the study is on factors which affect learning including financial incentives, individual ability, organizational norms and constraints, training, and the social environment. The most important result of the study indicates that individual learning can be aggregated into organizational learning, and the latter can thus be measured explicitly. Also the study of learning can help any organization build a quantitative description of learning within the organization's workforce. Also the developed learning maps may help management to better understand the diversity of its workforce.

In this chapter we cover eight diverse papers on management issues of interest to health care institutions. Application of the results can benefit any organization to improve its operations, lower costs, and improve quality.

13.1 FOCUSSING IN HEALTH CARE ORGANIZATIONS

Organizations that provide professional services and are focused on serving a particular market segment or segments benefit from competitive advantages over non-focused organizations. The advantages derive from being able to design a service delivery system that is fully concentrated on the needs of the segment(s) that the organization is focused on serving. In particular, economies of atmosphere are obtained, defined as the joint positive impact of a distinct set of values, (tacit) knowledge, and competencies on the technical efficiency of the firm. Focusing is a competitive strategy decision by the firm. In focusing, the firm designs the service process and infrastructure to meet the needs of the specific market segments. It might lead to standardization or customization in the service operations, depending on the needs of the customers. There is very little information on how managers should make focusing decisions, particularly in the health care industry. This paper addresses that gap in information.

Two of the researchers, Curtis McLaughlin and Shitao Yang, are from the Kenan-Flagler School of Business at the University of North Carolina, and the third researcher, Roland van Dierdonck, is from the Vlerick School of Management, University of Ghent, Belgium (1995). They worked to develop a framework to assist managers in professional services on how to make focusing decisions. They used three sources of data from the health care industry to support such as framework:

1. industry statistics,
2. case studies, and
3. questionnaire surveys.

The researchers evaluated the advantages and disadvantages of focusing on outpatient surgery centers as the primary example for the paper. Their primary data came from questionnaire surveys completed by ambulatory surgery unit managers. The researchers then contrasted the differences and similarities of the operational processes between outpatient surgery centers and traditional surgical settings in hospitals.

Outpatient surgery centers (OSCs) are focused on elective (schedulable) surgeries. The degree of focus for a particular OSC may range from specializing in a single type of surgery to providing more general, wider varieties of surgeries. There are up to five ways on which to base the focus of an OSC:

1. customer group,
2. service concept,
3. operating strategy or process,
4. service area or site, and
5. group of providers.

The main decision process in setting up an OSC is: 1. what set of surgeons and their patients to seek and what range of services to provide, and 2. how to organize the service to best meet customer needs. In making these decisions, managers need to assess the competitive strategy for the organization, what the core competencies of the organization are intended to be, what kind of processes they will need to carry out to provide value-added services, and how to maximize efficiency in the service delivery system.

The researchers contrasted the differences between OSCs and traditional surgery settings in hospitals, where patients are confronted with different operating processes and conflicting priorities. The advantages of focusing in the OSC in terms of operational efficiency and patient (customer) and staff satisfaction over the traditional (non-focused) setting are pointed out. The researchers contrasted the two settings based on fifteen different questions. These fifteen questions form the framework on which the researchers suggest managers use to make focusing decisions. The framework considers the segmentation alternatives, how the process would need to be adapted, the benefits and disadvantages to combining or not combining segments, processes or value-added activities, and what should be the final service delivery system configuration.

While focusing may cause an organization to lose economies of scope and scale, these losses can sometimes be superseded by other economies, such as fewer support staff, less capital investment or greater market penetration in the focused segment(s) due to better service. The researchers showed that by focusing, OSCs are successful in significantly reducing capital and other costs which allows them to meet the reduced scale and scope of operations in a cost-effective manner.

The outcome of the study provides a valuable framework of questions and considerations to help managers make focusing decisions in professional service organizations. While some of the questions may be obvious, the complete list is comprehensive, and therefore, if used, would avoid overlooking some important considerations. While the list was developed within the health care sector and in particular focused on outpatient surgery centers, more research would need to be done to determine how well it applies as a general framework for other industries.

13.2   ANALYSIS OF NURSING HOME OUTCOMES

This paper describes an investigation of the attributes of the residents, the facilities and the long-term outcomes of nursing home patients. The researchers, Frank Porell, Francis G. Caro, Ajith Silva, and Mark Monane (1998) decided to analyze certain long-term health outcomes of patients in nursing home settings. The authors performed a longitudinal analysis of resident and facility attributes associated with multiple nursing home outcomes.

The nursing homes that were studied are located in Massachusetts. Their data was taken from quarterly reports used in their Medicaid reimbursement systems. This data assisted the researchers in creating patient histories ranging in length from three months to three years for patients in over 500 nursing home facilities. Person-level statistical models were estimated for four health outcomes to identify factors associated with changes in resident health outcomes over time. The study explores the construct validity of statistical models, derived from administrative data, relating health outcomes to both resident risk factors and to the structural attributes of nursing homes.

The data used was primarily taken from the Management Minutes Questionnaire (MMQ). The MMQ determines the case-mix reimbursement to nursing homes in the state of Massachusetts. The data on the MMQ is collected from information contained in a resident's clinical record including a licensed nursing summary, daily licensed nursing notes, physician's orders and progress notes, activities of daily living (ADL) flow sheets, medication administration records, treatment records, and care plans.

The sample size of nursing home residents consisted of 4,438 patients. The data collected for these patients helped to create the patient histories. The ADL status items were each specified as a simple dichotomy of independence versus dependence. The researchers defined dependence as either including the assistance of staff members, total dependence, or the formal reception of restorative services. The researchers also measured the mental health of the patients. This was specified as either behavioral problems or memory impairment. Another variable measured was incontinence. This was classified as either regular bladder or bowel incontinence or occasional incontinence. The sample means of the outcome measures suggest a relatively frail, but durable elder resident population. In addition, sensitivity analyses were also performed to test for potential biases associated with the use of data with left-truncated residence histories.

The results show that the more fragile Medicaid patients showed quicker deterioration in ADL functional status than similar patients who show the same demographic and clinical conditions. The results also show that the older a patient is, the quicker the decline, when compared to similar patients who have the same condition. In addition, aside from state-dependence effects, significant positive coefficients for the ADL and incontinence variables suggest that more physically impaired residents were at greater risk for increased cognitive and behavioral problems. The findings of the study show that the residents with mental dysfunctions showed a greater decline when compared with similar patients.

This study has several implications for business, especially in the health care management field. Nursing home administrators can utilize this study to monitor the quality of health care to all residents, both Medicaid and self-pay. In addition, this study can assist practitioners in dealing with their nursing home patients. It can help them to determine whether the patients are normal under regular circumstances.

13.3   RESOURCE UTILIZATION IN HEALTH CARE

Case management (CM) is a method of organizing a fragmented group of health care service providers at the point of service delivery and includes acute, primary, and community settings. This can range from a simple referral to coordination between multiple providers. Considered an important component of care in many health care settings, the utility of CM is based more on its face value than on scientifically documented success. What do case managers do with what types of clients? What are the outcomes? What activity is associated with nursing home placement or hospitalization? These questions are examined in this study published by *Health Care Financing Review* authored by Robert Newcomer and Pamela Arnsberger, of the University of California, San Francisco, along with Xiulan Zhang, of the University of California, Berkeley (1999).

Chart data was used in this exploratory retrospective study. A probability sample of 893 cases from eight geographically dispersed sites, all part of the Medicare Alzheimer's Disease Demonstration project, was used in order to delineate CM activity. Client and caregiver (spouse, relative, or neighbor, for example) characteristics were partially obtained from interviews with the primary caregivers. Tracking of service use outcomes was obtained six months after CM was begun for each client, in order to look at the relationship between different types of CM actions with service use outcomes. Statistical analyses also used data from the Medicare Alzheimer's Disease Demonstration Evaluation (MADDE) and included principal factor analysis, odds-ratios, and logistics regression.

Case Manager Activities

42 "pure" types of CM activities were identified, grouped into the following categories:

1. routine service monitoring, including routine assessments and care plan development;
2. caregiver training/mental health approach, including the provision of disease management information to the caregiver;
3. crisis intervention, including referrals to adult protective services;
4. clinical nursing/caregiver support, including involvement by registered nurses;
5. caregiver empowerment/advocacy approach, including assistance in obtaining social services; and,
6. client health and placement approach, consisting mainly of discharge planning and placement assistance.

Case Manager Activities as Related to Client and Caregiver Characteristics

Certain results were not meaningful due to the fact that all members of the sample had Alzheimer's. Other relationships, however, were evident, some of which were: 1. limitations in typical client activities of daily living (ADLs) were positively associated with routine monitoring; and 2. depression, an assumed risk factor among caregivers, was found to be significantly negatively related to routine monitoring and positively related to discharge planning and placement assistance.

Case Manager Activities and Service Use Outcomes

A stronger pattern emerged here than in the previous analysis. Service use outcomes included nursing services, nursing home placement, and hospital placement as well as home-based benefits such as companion care, homemaker use, and personal care. Three CM activities were significantly related to health care use:

1. routine monitoring was associated with a lower likelihood of nursing home use;
2. clinical nursing was associated with a lower rate of hospital admissions; and,
3. discharge planning and placement assistance was associated with more hospital use.

Other findings included: routine monitoring was significantly and positively related to the home-based outcomes, as well as with nursing services; and clinical nursing and caregiver support, along with caregiver empowerment, reduced the likelihood of homemaker services.

Business implications

Effective resource utilization is a key issue for managed care organizations. However, the relative role played by case managers versus other providers in managed care is not widely understood. By clarifying CM activities, studies such as this can be used to improve staffing, treatment protocols, and client service outcomes. Although further research is required, the clinical nursing factor appeared to have a protective association against the likelihood of hospitalization. Also, the inverse relationship between routine monitoring and nursing home placement was significant.

13.4   ENTREPRENEURIAL FAILURE AND SUCCESS

Entrepreneurship is desired and valuable to society. Yet, failure is often pervasive. Theories currently reflect an equally pervasive antifailure bias. When this is done the inherent risk involved in entrepreneurial ventures is often minimized. Social norm encourages risk taking as long as the risk taker does not lose. Basically, the tendency to view failure negatively introduces a pervasive bias in the entrepreneurship theory and research.

Researcher Rita Gunther McGrath (1999) of Columbia University decided to characterize entrepreneurial initiatives as real options whose value is fundamentally influenced by uncertainty. In an attempt to show how an option can reveal the conditions under which an antifailure bias can hinder understanding of the systematic relationship between success and failure, leading to negative consequences. Real options reasoning allows more of a failure's possible benefits to be captured and the most egregious of its costs to be contained. She applies these ideas at the economy and firm levels. The objective is to offer ideas that might help redirect the theoretical focus in entrepreneurship from a preoccupation with achieving success and avoiding failure to a more integrated view of how the two phenomena are related.

McGrath defined the entrepreneurial processes as the set of activities through which innovation can integrate existing combinations of factors of production in both manufacturing and service sectors. The entrepreneurial initiative is stated as a specific effort by a new combination of resources. Failure of the initiative is termination as a result of falling short of intended goals. She used the real options theory that concerns classes of investments in real assets that are similar to financial options in structure. It is because of the advantages it has over conventional approaches under conditions of uncertainty.

This study includes discussion about entrepreneurial initiatives as real options, real options in bundles indicating that there are interrelated effects to evaluate when attempting to describe what leads to the success or failure of the entrepreneurial process. Also discussed are entrepreneurial initiatives and wealth creation and the impact on the economy and firms. The researcher addressed antifailure bias by extrapolating to the future from past success, cognitive biases, and direct manipulation. These reasonings are utilized in an attempt to minimize failure without taking into account what is beneficial about the process of failure. The study includes a detailed table using examples of unintended consequences of an antifailure bias.

The researcher stated that normally lowering of variance is utilized to reduce failure. The study introduces five propositions to increase the variance of an opportunity. The opportunity was directly related to the slack. The remaining propositions discuss the implications of passivity given that potential failure discourages entrepreneurship by penalizing those who try and holding blameless those who do not try at all.

The researcher discusses several implications of real options reasoning including the provision of the conceptual foundation for a new perspective on the dynamics of performance, survival, and choice in entrepreneurship. The research can be applied by linking the positive and negative outcomes to a systematic measure to explain economic values and uncertainty when failure occurs in the entrepreneurial process. Failure is easier to explain whereas the reasons for success include more variables. Performing a failure analysis can be a powerful tool for resolving uncertainty of an entrepreneurial venture.

The important point the researcher addresses is that it matters relatively little if numerous inexpensive options expire (ventures fail), provided that returns are substantial for one or more of the surviving ventures.

The researcher concludes with the point that carefully analyzing failures, instead of celebrating successes, can be very beneficial to future ventures. In other words when one acquires options, not every option is expected to be utilized. The majority are expected to expire. Analogously, entrepreneurial activities are not expected to all be successful. Some will be successes, but many others will be terminated before excessive losses are incurred.

13.5   DECISION MAKING BY HEALTH SERVICES MANAGERS

When making decisions, are managers more likely to optimize the decision or satisfy the requirements? Optimizing a decision is either maximizing the benefits or minimizing the costs or a combination of the two alternatives. Even though managers may be facing similar decisions the model that they view the problem through will make outcomes vary. Recent research has shown that to understand a manager's decision making process you must understand the model that they apply to the process of decision making.

Clinical Psychologist John Ormrod, of De Monfort University of Leicester (1993), performed a series of interviews with sixteen managers employed by the National Health Service. His testing is concerned with examining the criteria that underlie the decision making process.

John Ormrod's research consisted of a three-stage process. The first stage consisted of an interview with all 16 managers discussing the strategic decisions that they are currently facing. Along with these decisions he also explored the factors (criteria, constructs) that the managers used to make these decisions. The data collected was used to create grids with the decisions and criteria representing elements of the grid. Stage two of the process consisted of individual interviews with seven of the managers. At these interviews they discussed the current strategic dilemmas that they face. They also looked at the factors that they individually are using during their decision making process. The subjects then rated each of these factors in order of importance. Grids were established and visually analyzed. Two of the seven managers were re-interviewed one month afterwards to see how the process of examining their decision-making has affected them. The last stage consisted of collecting grids for five of the subjects using problems at a more mundane level.

As stated by the author the results are not presented as hard facts but rather reflections and interpretations of the researcher. With this stated we can look at some of the results that the author has derived from the experiment. During stages one and two the subjects could recall between two and six strategic decisions that they are currently facing. Between nine and twenty-four factors were determined as those that influence their decision-making. The number of factors however, does not equate directly to the complexity of the decision making process used. After analysis it was determined that in some cases there was little variation on how each of the criteria were being applied to the decision at hand. Some interesting criteria trends were also present after analysis. Eighty-seven percent of the subjects indicated "political factor" as important while only thirty percent viewed "quality" and "vision" as important. Generally political factors are viewed as immediate or short-term factors while the others are more long term in nature.

There was also the presence of "emotional" factors brought up by many of the subjects. Criteria such as "keeping people happy," "honesty," "loyalty," and "pleasing others" were said to influence their decision making. This goes against the heartless manager stereotype. The level of stress that a manager is under was also shown to affect their decision-making. The higher the stress the manager is under the lesser the number of criteria used to make decisions. Basically they get into an increased level of satisfying versus optimization.

The last result came from the two managers that were re-interviewed after the second stage of the experiment. Both managers felt that they now viewed the process with an increased number of criteria in mind. In fact one actually created the grid for the factors that he was using.

This study helps confirm that decisions being made by managers are intended to satisfy the requirements versus optimize the results. Many managers are making decisions with very narrow and focused criteria. These criteria are generally satisfying the short-term goals, which may not be an optimizing decision for the long term. By understanding the process it can be used to benefit the business world today. Companies could implement a simple training exercise to look at the factors that their managers are using to make decisions. By doing so they would then be able to give the managers the insight into the process along with some tools needed to widen their criteria to optimize more of their decisions. This learned point and solution will perhaps begin to improve the decisions being made in organizations today.

13.6   WORK RELATIONSHIPS OF PHYSICIANS WITH HOSPITALS

Strategies of vertical integration are increasingly being used by hospitals to link community physicians and embed them in the organization. Such strategies are ultimately intended to address problems of access, cost, and quality. Currently there are three basic models for embedding physicians in organizations: autonomous, or voluntary participation; conjoint, or contractual relationships; and heteronomous, or hospital ownership of the practice with hospital-based salaries for physicians. Mixed evidence exists that physician-hospital integration yields benefits for either side. In their study, Lawton R. Burns, Stephen M. Shortell, and Ronald M. Andersen (1998) address this issue, in *Research in the Sociology of Health Care*, Volume 15.

Description of study

The study analyzes the effect of two types of physician-hospital integration on work relationships with physicians. The work relationship is then examined in terms of its effect on physician attitudes and admitting behaviors. The first type of integration concerns economic linkage in the form of hospital-based practice settings, salaried employment, joint ventures and heavy in-patient utilization. Administrative involvement is the second type of physician-hospital integration and includes: board role, executive role, and committee role. Four dimensions of perceived physician-hospital work relationships were developed:

1. autonomy, or hospital respect for physician autonomy;
2. voice, or physician participation in decision-making;
3. commitment, or physician commitment to the primary hospital; and
4. trust, or physician trust in the primary hospital.

The study was conducted in 1990 and was principally based on results of a survey administered to 6,814 physicians.

Results

After eliminating those who had moved, retired, or died, the final respondent sample total consisted of 2,320 physicians who practiced in 90 different hospitals. A physician sub-sample of 1,671 physicians represents those with economic joint-venture arrangements with hospitals. Another 1,400 physician sub-sample reflects those for whom admitting data was available. The following results represent statistically significant findings.

Economic linkage

On average, physicians were found to spend 18 percent of their practice time in hospital-based practice and derive one-quarter of their income from salaried employment. Linkage time with the primary hospital was 19 years on average, and approximately three-quarters of a physician's admissions were to the physician's primary hospital. A slight decrease in physician admitting volume and loyalty was evident, which reflects the historical decline nationwide in hospital admissions and the shift of allegiances due to hospital integration efforts and managed care contracting. Physicians who spend more time in hospital-based roles tended to report more favorable evaluations on all four quality-of-relationship dimensions. Physicians who derive more income from salaried payments reported more favorably in all dimensions except autonomy. Duration of linkage was associated with favorable evaluation of voice and commitment.

Administrative involvement

Less than 10 percent of physicians were found to occupy board roles, roughly 25 percent occupied executive roles, and nearly 13 percent performed committee roles. Physicians in governance and executive roles reported more favorably regarding all or most work relationship dimensions. Physicians in committee roles reported more favorably in respect to voice and commitment. Decision-making voice and organizational commitment were found to be positively influenced by both economic linkage and administrative involvement, while trust appeared to be influenced by economic linkage and involvement in governance. Physicians in joint ventures reported more positively in terms of voice, commitment, and trust.

Admitting behavior

Admission loyalty exerted a positive affect on commitment and trust, and admission volume positively affected commitment.

Implications for health care organizations

Physicians expressing greater commitment to the hospital are likely to maintain or increase their percentage of total admissions over time. None of the other three work relationship variables exerted significant effects. Economic linkage and administrative involvement exert few direct or inconsistent effects on admitting behavior over time. Some economic linages (e.g., salaried positions) weaken admitting loyalty while others (e.g., hospital-based roles) strengthen it. There is no evidence that salaried roles either increase or decrease admitting volume (productivity). Over time, there is some weak evidence that economic integration and favorable work relationships between physicians and hospitals may reinforce one another. Economic linkage can improve certain work relationships, which promote more admitting behavior to the primary hospital.

13.7 LEARNERS AND ORGANIZATIONAL LEARNING

Manufacturers face increasing competition in their field. In response to the competition, they must know how to efficiently use their resources. Understanding their organizational learning pattern is one method to provide them important information to wisely utilize their work force and increase production. Implications from this study clearly impact health care organizations with their labor-intensive activities.

Many factors, financial incentives, individual variability, individual ability, organizational norms and constraints, training, and the nature of the social environment affect learning. Learning and improvement also occur in different collections of people, such as in teams, and work groups.

To measure learning the researchers Uzumeri and Nembhard (1998) obtained a large data base from a large U.S. manufacturer. The data base contained work performance records on nearly 4,000 learning episodes based on assembly tasks. The data was collected electronically at each work station with bar-code readers and timing devices.

Each work performance record represented a task. These tasks were then classified by the company's industrial engineers. There were 119 different tasks, each task containing numerous learning episodes. The overall data base contained nearly 68,000 individual performance records.

The researchers then attempted to fit the data to a variety of statistically-based learning curves, which were then plotted and compared.

The results of the study revealed a variety of learning patterns of regularity and variance. Applications of their method include:

1. integration of learning into product costing,
2. use of learning maps to gauge training effectiveness, and
3. comparison of learning maps for facility flows, facility location, and facility investment decisions.

The most important result indicates that individual learning can be aggregated into organizational learning, and the latter can thus be measured explicitly. This result is important because up till now learning curves have focused on individuals or individual processes.

In conclusion, the learning application can help any organization build a quantitative description of learning within its workforce. The maps may help management to better understand the diversity of their workforce. Shifts in the distribution of the parameter estimates may help managers to identify when external forces are impacting the learning performance. Comparisons of successive maps may indicate if learning is accelerating or eroding and whether the ultimate prospects for performance are increasing or decreasing. Comparison of maps across operation units may reveal differences in learning behavior in different locations, at dissimilar tasks, at a different time or among workers with different types and levels of training.

REFERENCES

Burns, L. R., Shortell, S. M., & Anderson, R. M. (1998). Does familiarity breed contentment?: Attitudes and behaviors of integrated physicians. *Research in the Sociology of Health Care, 15*, 85-110.

McGrath, R. G. (1999). Falling forward: Real options reasoning and entrepreneurial failure. *The Academy of Management Review, 24*(1), 13-30.

McLaughlin, C. P., Yang, S., & van Dierdonck, R. (1995). Professional service organizations and focus. *Management Science, 41*(7), 1185-1193.

Newcomer, R., Arnsberger, P., & Zhang, X. (1999). Case management, client risk factors, and service use. *Health Care Financing Review, 19*(1), 105-120.

Ormrod, J. (1993). Decision making in health service managers. *Management Decision, 31*(7), 8-14.

Porell, F., Caro, F. G., Silva, A., & Monane, M. (1998). A longitudinal analysis of nursing home outcomes. *Health Services Research, 33*(4), 835.

Uzumeri M., & Nembhard, D. (1998). A population of learners: A new way to measure organizational learning. *Journal of Operations Management, 16*, 515-528.

CHAPTER 14

STRATEGIC MANAGEMENT IN HEALTH SYSTEMS

This chapter covers management strategy and its implications for the general and overall future and economic health of health institutions in general and hospitals in particular.

The first study focuses on governing board structure, business strategy, and performance of acute care hospitals. The central theme of the study is based on the board members' ability to contribute to strategic and policy decisions depending in part on their occupational background. The database consisted of the board members of over one hundred acute care hospitals. Results of the study revealed that organizational size was the only variable related to strategy. Board composition depended on the strategy typology of a hospital. Two main strategy types of hospitals were identified. They were prospectors and defenders. A hospital with a defender strategy offers a limited amount of services and maintains market position through internal efficiency. A hospital with a prospector strategy is the opposite of a defender and emphasizes the gathering and use of external information. The results revealed that prospectors had the largest and most heterogeneous board. Defenders had the smallest and most homogeneous board. Also prospectors had few medical staff members on their board, while defenders had the largest number of staff members on their boards. The

Proven Solutions for Improving Health and Lowering Health Care Costs, pages 201–213.
Copyright © 2003 by Information Age Publishing, Inc.
All rights of reproduction in any form reserved.
ISBN: 1-59311-000-6 (paper), 1-59311-001-4 (cloth)

results point to the importance of board structure for the future health of the affected institutions.

The second study examines conflict in top management teams and asks the question if it affects performance. Top management teams from 48 firms in the food processing industry were surveyed. Members of the teams were questioned regarding the decisions in which they had participated. The results of the study indicated that higher levels of cognitive (functional) conflict will produce higher quality decisions and higher levels of affective (dysfunctional) acceptance and understanding. Also higher levels of affective conflict will produce lower quality decisions with lower levels of affective acceptance and understanding. The conclusion is that conflict is good for strategic decision-making provided it is only cognitive and not affective.

The third study asks how new firms can increase their chances of survival. The study was based on a sample of over 100 firms in the computer industry. The one surprising result of the research is that competitive conditions are not related to the mortality of young firms. The implication of the study is that founders of new firms have two ways of improving their firms' chances of survival. Rapidly rising demand in an industry is one way to improve survival. Another strategy for survival is the rapid acquisition of resources in specialized markets through direct acquisition or mergers.

The fourth study explores the benefits of formal strategic networks among small and medium-sized companies (SMEs). The authors investigated whether SMEs provide net benefits or net costs to the SME member firms, and they tried to find out what factors produce these net benefits or costs. The study consisted of a case-type study. Only two SME networks were studied and both were in the wood products industry. The results indicated that net gains are realized by SME member firms. Homogeneous networks experienced a high degree of both positive transactional and transformational outcomes. More heterogeneous networks experienced positive transactional benefits but few transformational benefits. The overall conclusion was that SME networks are beneficial to SMEs.

The fifth study describes an analysis of the rationale for and consequence of non-profit and for-profit ownership conversions. The database consisted of 33 non-profit to for-profit hospital conversions and 50 for-profit to non-profit hospital conversions over a four-year period. The results revealed that hospitals that convert are more likely to have experienced a financial loss prior to conversion, and are more likely to be located in an urban market. Following conversion average revenues increased associated with an increase in operating expenses. Conversion was reasonably successful because only 3 hospitals of each type of conversion closed during the study period.

The sixth study explored differentiation and agglomeration in the Manhattan hotel industry. The researchers' main opposing themes were that new hotels will locate far from similar established hotels to minimize local competition, or new hotels will locate close to similar established hotels to benefit from agglomeration economies. The research partially supported the researchers themes. Hotels tended to locate farther away from similar hotels against whom they could not offer specific advantages in either size, price, service, facilities or image. Yet hotels with characteristics similar to those of their competitors located close to competing hotels. These hotels intended to invade a competing hotel's niche with some superior characteristics.

The seventh and final study addressed privatization and productivity. The question posed was: does privatization increase productivity? The researchers studied 41 companies that were privatized from 15 different countries. The results of their study showed that results were generally improved. For the 41 firms in the study, average return on sales after privatization increased by approximately 2 percentage points, debt doubled and employment increased by 20 percent. The fear of downsizing by many employees did not occur but considerable restructuring of operations did occur. The results also show that changing the chief executive officer profoundly influences performance in newly privatized firms.

In this chapter we have explored a number of areas where strategic management decisions have made profound changes in the organization. Strategic management decisions can have considerable impact on the performance of organizations provided they are made by and supported by a large segment of the organization. Strategic decisions imposed by the upper management group only will face considerable difficulty in being accepted and implemented, if at all.

14.1 RELATIONSHIP OF BOARD STRUCTURE, BUSINESS STRATEGY, AND PERFORMANCE

Traditionally, hospital governing boards served mainly as community stewards and were not actively involved in the strategic management of the hospital. As the hospital industry has experienced increasing environmental pressures however, governing boards are being asked to become more involved in strategic and policy decisions. In order for the board to be successful in this activity, it must be instructed to complement the overall strategy of the hospital. This study examined the relationship between board structure and hospital strategy based on the financial performance of the hospital.

Gary Young, from the Agency for Health Care Policy and Research, Rafik Beekun, from the University of Nevada, and Gregory Ginn, from the University of Central Texas (1992), conducted a survey based on Miles' and Snow's topology of business strategy to study the issue. The central theme of the study was based on the board members' ability to contribute to strategic and policy decisions depending in part on their occupational background. The survey solicited information on board size, occupational diversity, and medical staff representation of 109 acute care hospitals. In addition, the survey asked the respondent to identify whether it employed a prospector, analyzer, defender, or reactor business strategy. The authors hypothesized that the comparative size, diversity, and number of medical staff members on the governing board will each be a function of the hospital's strategy. A fourth hypothesis tested the financial performance of the hospital as a function of the relationship between strategy and board structure.

A defender strategy was defined as offering a limited amount of services and maintaining market position by stressing internal efficiency. The prospector is the opposite of a defender, and emphasizes the gathering and use of external information. The analyzer strategy is a combination of the defender and prospector strategies, and relies on both internal and external information. The reactor strategy is often viewed as a non-strategy, and has no consistent response to the environment.

Data for the strategy topology of the study was collected through a mailed questionnaire directed to the chief executive officer of 370 acute care hospitals in Pennsylvania and New York states; 109 usable responses resulted. Data relating to board size and composition was obtained from the American Hospital Association special survey on hospital governance; data on organizational size and system membership were obtained from the AHA Guide to the Health Care Field. Financial performance data were obtained from Medicare cost reports. The independent variable for analysis was organizational strategy, with covariates of organizational size and system membership. The dependent variables were board size, diversity, and medical staff representation.

Univariate ANCOVAs, a form of analysis of variance, were used to test the first three hypotheses. The fourth hypothesis (relating to financial performance) was tested using a complicated multi-step statistical process. Four high performers were randomly identified for each of the four strategy categories based on the hospital's return on assets. The mean of each category in relation to the three structural attributes was calculated, and a score was determined. A multiple regression analysis was used to assess the relationships between the scores and financial performance. Control variables included physicians per capita, proportion of population over 65 years of age, number of hospital beds in proportion to total number of beds in the market, and per capita income.

Results of the study indicated that all four of the defined strategies were significantly related to all three structural attributes, but that organizational size was the only covariate significantly related to strategy; system membership was insignificant. Prospectors had the largest board; defenders had the smallest. Prospectors had the most heterogeneous governing boards, while defenders had the most homogeneous. Prospectors had the smallest proportion of medical staff members on the board, and defenders had the largest. These results are consistent with the different strategy emphases, and results were also consistent for the two remaining strategies. With respect to financial performance, a greater match between board structure and system strategy affected hospital financial performance in a direct relationship, although this relationship was limited.

The results of this study help to better understand the possible relationships between board structure and business strategy. Most of the research on board structure to date has examined organizational size and system membership as the main influencing factors of board structures; this study outlines the importance of business strategy in the mix. This is important in that many policy proposals are targeted to improving hospital performance, and may have otherwise overlooked this important variable.

14.2   CONFLICT IN MANAGEMENT TEAMS: DOES IT REALLY IMPROVE STRATEGIC TEAM PERFORMANCE?

For many top management teams the quality, consensus, and effective acceptance of key decisions are crucial components for maintaining their high corporate performance. Group interaction techniques introduce intentional conflict into these strategic discussions to improve decision quality through the diversity of their members. While improving quality this cognitive team decision and the effect it has on the quality, consensus, and acceptance of these decisions are explored.

High quality decisions are a necessity for any organization, but these decisions may be tempered by a lack of full group consensus and acceptance. Top management teams often consist of numerous diverse individuals whose wide-ranging experiences and capabilities lead to innovative, high-quality decisions. Through the development of these decisions, the management teams utilize various interaction methods to arrive at their decisions, with the most effective of these methods typically involving some form of critical debate of the opposing positions. These methods, of which devil's advocacy (DA) and dialectical inquiry (DI) are two, focus the individuals on opposite sides of the issues through the use of cognitive (functional) conflict, with the person who originated the idea of "defending" the position from the "attack" of others. As a by-product of this cognitive conflict, affective (dysfunctional) conflict may often arise, usually when the cognitive conflict is perceived as personal criticism. This affective portion of conflict hampers the consensus and acceptance of the group and can reduce the ability to effectively implement the high-quality decisions. This introduction of conflict creates "watered-down" results.

Top management teams will use cognitive conflict to help produce their high-quality decisions, while realizing that affective conflict may result and can soften the implementation effects. These teams have placed themselves precariously on the fine line separating high-quality decisions, with lower consensus and acceptance from the team members, and low-quality decisions, with high consensus and acceptance from the members.

Allen C. Amason (1996) from Mississippi State University, recently examined the issue at top management teams from the food-processing and furniture industries. Amason surveyed forty-eight firms in these industries from across the United States, with the top management teams being questioned regarding decisions in which they had participated. For each firm, Amason contacted the chief executive officer and asked each to describe the most recent strategic decision and provide the names of the managers making that decision. The actual survey was then sent to each of those team members responsible for that strategic decision. Amason attempted to measure both cognitive and affective conflict in these teams, and their respective effects on the quality, understanding, commitment, and acceptance of the management team decisions.

The direct results of the study indicate that higher levels of cognitive conflict will produce higher quality decisions and higher levels of affective acceptance, while higher levels of affective conflict will produce lower quality decisions with lower levels of affective acceptance. The outcome also shows that higher levels of cognitive conflict will produce a high level of decision understanding, while higher levels of affective conflict will not produce lower levels of decision understanding. The study also suggests that higher levels of cognitive conflict will not produce higher levels of commitment, while higher levels of affective conflict will not produce lower levels of commitment.

The end result of this study reveals that conflict acts as a double-edged sword, with the cognitive edge producing the higher levels of quality and acceptance and the affective producing lower levels of quality and acceptance. In attempting to stimulate the functional conflict for quality, the management teams may be inadvertently introducing the dysfunctional conflict which erodes the team itself. Top management teams must attempt to harness the power of cognitive conflict while restraining the negative impact of affective conflict. By doing so, the management teams will reap the benefits of high-quality decisions which will provide the continued success in the implementation of these decisions and the ultimate success of the firm.

14.3   HOW CAN NEW FIRMS INCREASE THEIR CHANCES OF SURVIVAL?

Market demand is the primary environmental influence on young-firm survival likelihoods, according to Professor Elaine Romanelli of Duke University (1989). Specialist organizations have a higher likelihood of surviving their early years than generalists, aggressive organizations have a greater chance of early survival than efficient firms, generalist strategies improve survival likelihoods when sales are increasing, and more efficient organizations will fare better when sales are declining.

New organizations are notoriously poor at surviving their early years. Some investigators have examined the effects of environmental conditions on rates of death among new organizations, while others have emphasized the characteristics and activities of organizations as determinants of young firms' mortality. Romanelli's is the first study to explore the separate and combined influences of environmental conditions (resource availabilities and competitive concentration) and organizational strategies (market breadth and market aggressiveness) on survival likelihood of young firms.

Romanelli first distinguishes between firms that operate in broad or multiple market segments and firms that operate in narrow or few segments. Specialization is particularly suitable for young firms because it typically requires the expenditure of fewer resources than generalism, and also helps a new organization establish a foothold in the marketplace that is relatively free of competition from larger organizations. However, when demand for a product or service is increasing and competitive concentration is declining, a more general approach to exploiting market resources may also be appropriate for new firms. In these conditions venture capital can fuel a young organization's entry to multiple market segments, and young organizations can compete in the general marketplace on a relatively equal footing.

Romanelli also distinguishes between firms that are quick and aggressive to pursue newly available resources and those that concentrate on the efficient use of existing resources. Aggressive firms risk the expenditure of resources to control additional resources, while efficient firms seek to protect an established position in the marketplace by husbanding scarce organization resources. On average, young organizations will increase their chances of survival when they take an aggressive posture toward resource acquisition. However, there may be times when external resources are simply too scarce for young firms to seek dominance, even in narrow market segments. When demand is declining and concentration is increasing, efficient organizations should have a higher likelihood of surviving.

Romanelli studied all firms that were founded in the United States to produce minicomputers between 1957 and 1981. This segment of the computer industry was chosen because a large amount of data existed concerning competitors, markets, and technologies, and also this segment underwent substantial change during the time period in terms of number and size of competitors, core technologies, and product/market applications. Of the 108 firms identified, 44 survived through 1981 and 64 were classified as failures.

The one surprising result of this research is that competitive conditions are unrelated to the mortality of young firms. Perhaps the finding is peculiar to the minicomputer population over this particular time period, or perhaps technological ferment improves the chances for young firms' survival, or perhaps the mortality of young organizations is predominantly influenced by the relative abundance of resources in the environment, independent of general competitive conditions.

The significant implication of this study is that founders of new firms have two ways of improving their firms' chances of survival. First, they can time founding to coincide with rapidly increasing sales in the industry. Second, they can tailor their resource-acquisition strategies to environmental conditions. Aggressive acquisition of resources in specialized markets should improve survival likelihoods except when industry sales are rapidly increasing or decreasing. When sales are increasing rapidly, an aggressive attack on multiple and/or general markets will significantly reduce the risk of failure. Finally, when sales are declining rapidly, an efficient exploitation of resources in specialized markets will prove most effective.

14.4 LET US UNITE FOR THE COMMON GOOD

Formation of formal strategic networks among small and medium-sized companies (SMEs) in the U.S. will likely produce more positive outcomes than negative ones, says Sherry E. Human and Keith G. Provan (1997). Benefits gained, they point out, can be either transactional—i.e. economic—or transformational—i.e. non-economic. In other words, an SME which participates in such a network stands to either improve its short term earnings or sales performance, or stands to improve the processes by which it carries on its business, which should improve performance over the long run.

Much research to date on strategic networks has been focused on those among large firms, rather than those among SMEs. Such SME networks are much more established in economies outside the U.S., particularly in Northern Italy and in Denmark. In the 1990s, however, the historically competitive and individualistic business climate in the U.S. has given way to an emergence of strategic alliances among SMEs. The key questions answered by Human and Provan are: 1. Do strategic networks provide net benefits or net costs to SME member firms? and 2. What factors produce these net benefits or costs?

The researchers found that, on balance, net gains are realized by SME member firms. They determined that networks where most firms are in the same or similar business—i.e. competitors—experienced a high degree of both positive transactional and transformational outcomes, whereas networks where firms vary widely in the type of business—i.e. manufacturers/ wholesalers/suppliers combinations—experienced positive transactional outcomes but few positive transformational outcomes. Typical positive transactional outcomes were: accessing new contacts or markets, increasing credibility or clout, and generating new product ideas. Typical transformational outcomes were: sharing technology with other members, referring business to other members, and viewing member competitors as potential resources.

The researchers further found that in networks with similar firms—or high domain similarity—there was a strong presence of a central administrative organization for the network, compared with networks with low domain similarity. This can be explained by the fact that high domain-similar networks are largely comprised of competitors, which need an intermediary body to foster cooperation. Low domain-similar networks take on more of a vertical integration approach, and do not require a strong intermediary presence. The authors refer to this distinction in network structure as the network-as-organization vs. the network-as-interaction. The latter form is generally viewed as preferable, where members exchange information more freely and directly.

The research was limited in that only two networks were studied, and both were in the same industry—wood products. Significant research and analysis, however, was done on this sample, where approximately 50 individuals, both inside and outside the networks, were contacted for qualitative and quantitative information.

Despite risks of network participation, including loss of proprietary information, and the opportunity cost of spending resources on network activity, the researchers conclude that formation of formal strategic networks among SMEs indeed produces net positive outcomes for networks both with and without high domain similarity among the member firms.

14.5 RATIONALE FOR NON-PROFIT AND FOR-PROFIT OWNERSHIP CONVERSIONS

This study examines precursors to private hospital conversion, both from non-profit status to for-profit status and from for-profit status to non-profit status. The study also examines the effect of hospital conversions on hospital profitability, efficiency, staffing, and the probability of closure. The sale of a non-profit hospital to a for-profit purchaser may contribute to a hospital's objectives or may be necessary due to its resource constraints. The effect of hospital conversions on hospitals' financial and operating performance is an empirical question rather than a theoretical one.

Researcher Tami L. Mark (1999) works as a Senior Research Economist at the MEDSTAT Group in Washington, D.C. Her research was partially based on Health Care Financing Administration's Medicare Cost Report database. Also, the American Hospital Association's (AHA) Annual Survey of Hospitals provided information on staffing and was used to verify data about ownership and discharges as reported by the Medicare Cost Reports (MCR).

The AHA data was merged with the MCR data using the hospital's name and county. The study for the effect of conversions consisted of the hospitals that submitted MCR data and engaged in private non-profit to for-profit conversions, or vice versa, during the period of 1989 to 1993. There were 33 non-profit to for-profit conversions and 50 for-profit to non-profit conversions in this time period. The comparison group consisted of approximately 3,800 acute care private hospitals that did not convert over the same period. Nine years of pooled time-series data were constructed for comparison hospitals in a manner comparable to those of the conversion sample. The final sample consisted of about 32,000 observations.

The financial variables examined included total profit margins, average inpatient Medicare costs per Medicare discharge, average operating expenses per inpatient-equivalent discharge, and average revenues per discharge. Staffing ratios were calculated per case mix-adjusted patient day. The number of closures was measured using the AHA Annual Survey of Hospitals, which lists hospital closures by year. HMO penetration was measured as the percentage of a market's population enrolled in HMOs based on data collected by Interstudy and included on the Area Resource File.

The descriptive statistics indicate that hospitals that convert are more likely to have experienced a financial loss prior to conversion than the average hospital. Also, greater conversion activity occurred in urban markets among non-profit hospitals. Another result was that conversion activity is more likely when hospital markets are more competitive.

Profit margins following conversion were found to increase. Both types of conversions were associated with an increase in operating expenditures, possibly because investment in hospital capital is increased. Average revenues increased after both types of conversions. Of the 33 hospitals that converted from non-profit to for-profit, three closed. Of the 50 hospitals that converted from for-profit to non-profit, three also closed.

This study has several implications on general business and hospital management. First, policymakers and regulators may need to weigh the risks of allowing a hospital to change ownership against the risk that a hospital will close if it does not convert. As this industry becomes more competitive and experiences greater pressure for cost containment, the transfer of assets that occurs through conversions may grow more frequent and may become a more important way to keep hospitals open and well maintained. Another implication of this study is that the improvement in a hospital's financial performance after a change in ownership may stem more from the acquiring hospital's better management and/or enhanced resources than from characteristics inherent in different ownership types. Management is the key as opposed to the business status.

14.6 DIFFERENTIATION AND AGGLOMERATION IN THE MANHATTAN HOTEL INDUSTRY

Entrepreneurs have found that organizations must make two crucial decisions: what products to sell and where to locate. According to Baum and Haveman (1997) cost structure and access to demand depend on product characteristics and geographic location. The main theme of their research revolved around two opposing hypotheses: new firms will locate 1. far from similar established firms to minimize localized competition, or 2. close to similar established firms to benefit from similar agglomeration economies.

The research partially supported each hypothesis. Firms tended to locate further away from similar competitors against whom they could offer no specific advantage in either size, price, service, facilities, or image. Yet firms with characteristics similar to those of their competitors did juxta-position themselves against competing firms. These firms based their location decision on their predicted success of invading a competitor's niche while possessing some superior characteristics. Thus, a mutually beneficial relationship was created as two very similar firms attracted business for each other as well as for themselves, with each one cashing in on their particular twist of a virtually identical product.

The researchers reviewed numerous studies in similar areas and considered Manhattan Hotel data from 1898-1990. They did extensive calculations involving means, standard deviations, minimums, maximums, and various correlations and variables to determine relationships of size distance, price distance, and geographic distance. These relationships almost exclusively determined where new hotels located and how they packaged their product.

This study provides an outline for understanding the product mix and location of local competitors. In Buffalo, New York, Home Depot, Chase Pitkin, and Builders Square, all direct competitors, attempted to remain as far apart from each other as possible to minimize localized competition. Yet Wegmans and Tops, also competitors in the supermarket field, are subscribing to the theory that they benefit from each other through agglomeration of economies. That is the spillover from one benefits the other and vice versa.

14.7 PRIVATIZATION AND AND PRODUCTIVITY

Many government agencies have privatized their enterprises. Privatization, the process by which state-owned enterprises are sold to the private sector, has become one of the most important business phenomena of the last 15 years. Does privatization increase productivity? Much debate has been generalized about whether privatization tends to enhance a firm's financial performance. The central research question was: What strategic decisions differentiated firms that recorded greater post-privatization performance improvement from firms that recorded little improvement?

Researchers William A. Andrews of Stetson University, and Michael Dowling of Paderborn University (1998) studied forty-one companies that were privatized from fifteen different countries. All samples in their study moved from public to private ownership. The study does attempt to enter the politically sensitive debate over whether firm performance is superior in private or public companies. The research identifies the strategic choices associated with performance improvement after privatization.

The database employed was the University of Georgia's Privatization Database. Three years of annual reports before privatization and three years of annual reports after privatization were solicited from each firm. The data measured from each of these reports were used against the researchers hypotheses. The hypotheses were:

1. Privatized firms that offer stock options will show more performance improvement than privatized firms that do not offer stock options.
2. Privatized firms that reduce employment will show improvement in performance.
3. Among privatized firms without large state ownership interests, firms that restructured financially by increasing debt will improve performance more than those that do not increase debt.
4. Privatized firms that change their CEO will improve performance more than privatized firms that do not change their CEO.

The results of these findings proved that stock options link the interests of owners and managers, thereby reducing agency costs and improved firm performance as opposed to those agencies that did not offer stock options. As hypothesized, among firms with little State ownership influence, increasing debt was associated with improved performance. The results also show that changing the chief agent, the CEO, profoundly influences performance in newly privatized firms. However, the finding suggests that worker displacement, one of the strongest objections to privatization, may not contribute to improved financial performance. This research failed to find evidence of performance improvement associated with downsizing. A possible explanation for this finding is that some downsizing may occur in the pre-privatization period during which the firms were being prepared for sale. Such an occurrence would mask some of the downsizing associated with privatization. The finding also suggested that no difference exists in employment reduction, with respect to operational restructuring between firms that remain governmentally controlled after privatization and those that do not. Employment is a highly sensitive topic in the privatized context, and it has been previously suggested that overstaffing is an agency cost associated with State-owned enterprises. The research team determined that further testing is needed with respect to downsizing.

For the 41 firms in this study the average return on sales after privatization increased by approximately 2 percent of sales compared to pre-privatization results. Debt approximately doubled for the average post-privatization firm, and employment increased 20 percent.

A critical implication is that many public servants are concerned with privatizing for fear of downsizing and being displaced. This research did not prove this. With the trend of Total Quality Management, many firms that are re-engineering and restructuring are keeping the experienced worker and are reassigning employees within the organization. Decreased employee morale is associated with downsizing and is linked to overall employee performance. Another critical finding was that firms that replaced their leaders and top management profoundly increased performance. In State-owned enterprises, the owner, the public, has virtually no managerial influence except through government agents, the appointed officials, whose interests in the firm may be subordinate to their superior's political objective. Therefore, from this finding, replacing the public top leaders after privatization will increase the firm's performance.

It appears that privatization will continue to be among the most influential business trends of the next decade.

REFERENCES

Amason, A. C. (1996). Distinguishing the effects of functional and dysfunctional conflict on strategic decision making: Resolving a paradox for top management teams. *Academy of Management Journal, 39*(1), 123-148.

Andrews, W. A., & Dowling, M. J. (1998). Explaining performance changes in newly privatized firms. *The Journal of Management Studies, 35*(5), 601-617.

Baum, J. A. C., & Haveman, H. A. (1997). Love they neighbor? Differentiation and agglomeration in the Manhattan hotel industry, 1898-1990. *Administrative Science Quarterly, 42*, 304-338.

Human, S. E., & Provan, K. G. (1997). An emergent theory of structure and outcomes in small-firm strategic manufacturing networks. *Academy of Management Journal, 40*(2), 368-400.

Mark, T. L. (1999). Analysis of the rationale for, and consequences of, non-profit and for-profit ownership conversions. *Health Services Research, 34*(1, Part 1), 83-101.

Romanelli, E. (1989). Environments and strategies of organization start-up: Effects on early survival. *Administrative Science Quarterly, 34*(3), 369-387.

Young, G., Beekun, R. I., & Ginn, G. O. (1992). Governing board structure, business strategy, and performance of acute care hospitals: A contingency perspective. *Health Services Research, 27*(4), 115-137.

CHAPTER 15

MANAGED HEALTH CARE

This chapter presents summaries of the research results of six studies on managed health care. Managed care grew rapidly starting in the early 1970s in response to federal funding for feasibility and planning studies and for implementation of health maintenance organizations.

The first study evaluates the effects of various health plans on the outcomes of hospitalization among elderly patients with congestive heart failure. The study classified the patient sample into six groups including managed care, traditional Medicare, Medicaid, commercial or private insurance, self pay, and others such as workers' compensation. The researchers found that Medicare managed care patients were much more likely to enter a hospital through an emergency room than patients in other groups. They also found that when controlling for age, sex, and comorbidity, there were no statistical differences in the risk of dying between the six groups. Also the differences between readmission rates of the six groups were not statistically significant.

The second study covered trends in managed care contracting among U.S. hospitals. Three types of hospitals were covered in the study, early contractors, recent contractors, and non-contractors of managed care. To determine why hospitals belonged to one of the three groups various factors were explored, including location, geographic region, type of ownership, multi-institutional affiliation, size, financial and operating

Proven Solutions for Improving Health and Lowering Health Care Costs, pages 215–228.
Copyright © 2003 by Information Age Publishing, Inc.
All rights of reproduction in any form reserved.
ISBN: 1-59311-000-6 (paper), 1-59311-001-4 (cloth)

performance, reimbursement, and continuum of care. The research revealed that urban and metro region hospitals formed the highest percentage of early contractors. Early contractors were also typically members of systems or alliances, were financially stable and offered a wider range of services. The results also suggested that recent and non-contractors had much in common while early contractors appeared quite different. Recent and non-contractors are predominantly rural, small in size, have lower case mix, and are financially weaker.

The third study addresses managing care, incentives, and information. Specifically, the researchers estimated how specific structures, incentives, and processes embodied in the management of care within the hospital, as well as external market factors, actually influence hospital resource consumption. The study sample consisted of 37 hospitals in seven different health systems located in the Western USA. The study offers some preliminary findings on how to promote hospital efficiencies such as developing payment arrangements under which the hospital assumes economic risk (capitation), intensifying management of care processes for specific health problems (care paths) and providing systematic information to physicians on resource consumption for the care of their patients. This study also found that peer reports had no significant effect on resource utilization. Coordination of care delivery lowered costs by 7-12 percent but product line management increased cost by 8-14 percent. Hospital-employed physicians also lowered costs but specialists and exclusive physician contracts raised costs by 6-12 percent.

The fourth study explored how business strategies promote cost-effective patient behavioral changes. The researchers compared resource utilization of both fee for service (FFS) and health maintenance organization (HMO) patients. Financial incentives utilized for HMO patients included use of a physician gatekeeper and co-payments for each office visit by patients. Organizational changes included charts for all HMO patients, educational appeals to practice cost-effective care, monitoring, feedback, and exception management. Three important findings were:

1. HMO influenced both patient and provider to use strategies to reduce care;
2. HMO care used fewer expenditures; and
3. HMO patients and FFS patients were not treated differently, thus reducing cost of FFS patients also.

Hence, managed care can achieve savings but the savings do not just accrue to HMO patients but also to FFS patients.

The fifth study asks why employees keep choosing the high-premium health care plan. The study was conducted at one employer over a two-year period. The useful sample consisted of 287 employees. Employees could choose from two health plans, one a high premium plan with 100 percent coverage and a low premium plan with 80 percent coverage. Both plans had similar out-of-pocket payments limits, but the high premium plan had higher average out of pocket cost, but, of course, lower risk. Risk avoiders, especially women, typically would select the high premium but lower risk plan.

The sixth study explored not managed care but managed competition, the purchasing of health care by large employers for their employees, also called value purchasing. Value purchasing of health care includes new organizational arrangements, financial incentives for employees, and the formation of a new relationship with health plans through the evaluation and monitoring of quality through procurement strategies such as competitive bidding and direct contracting. New organizational arrangements involved more cooperation between the finance, controller and human resource departments. Financial incentives for employees are typically based on company premium contribution only for the lowest cost plans. For other higher cost plans employees must cover the difference in the premiums. Formation of new relationships take on a variety of forms, but generally focus on identifying levels of quality, establishing standards, keeping employees informed and direct contracting with provider groups thus bypassing HMOs. Significant cost savings have been realized, but squeezing providers and HMOs too severely has also lowered quality of care and is raising dissatisfaction among employees.

In this chapter we have covered a variety of research studies in managed care. All studies generally point to lowering health care costs, but excessive cost containment pressure is also creating dissatisfaction among providers and also among the clients, who see service quality deteriorating.

15.1   MANAGED CARE AND OUTCOMES OF HOSPITALIZATION AMONG ELDERLY PATIENTS WITH CONGESTIVE HEART FAILURE

Since its introduction in the early 1970s, there has been widespread debate about the quality of care under managed care. This debate has intensified as more and more elderly patients have entered Medicare-managed care plans. Many contend that patient care suffers, while others believe that quality of care improves under managed care. Unfortunately, scientific research has been unable to settle the dispute. All research to date has produced conflicting results.

Researchers Hanyu Ni, Ph.D., Deirdre J. Nauman, RN, and Ray Hershberger, MD, (1998) from the Oregon State University studied all patients in the Oregon Hospital Discharge records who were 65 years of age or older and were diagnosed with congestive heart failure. They sought to test what impact health maintenance organizations-managed care membership had on quality of care outcomes for patients with congestive heart failure.

The researchers classified their sample of patients into six groups based on health insurance coverage. The groups were managed care, traditional Medicare, Medicaid, commercial or private insurance, self-pay, and other (workers compensation, division of health services). The outcome variables used by the researchers were type of admission, length of hospital stay, in-hospital mortality rate, and hospital re-admission with three months of discharge.

The researchers used multiple regression to determine the relationship between Medicare-managed care and length of hospital stay. They also developed a stepwise logistic regression model to determine the factors that contributed to in-hospital death. In addition, they used multiple logistic regression to determine the relationship between Medicare-managed care and in-hospital mortality rate, type of admission, and re-admission for congestive heart failure.

The researchers found that Medicare-managed care patients in the study were much more likely to enter the hospital through the emergency room than patients in the other insurance groups. They also discovered that lengths of stay of Medicare-managed care patients were slightly lower than those of other patients in the study. However, the group also found that when controlling for age, sex, and comorbidity, there were no statistical differences in the risk of dying between the six health insurance coverage groups. In addition, the authors discovered that differences between re-admission rates of the six insurance groups were not statistically significant.

Unfortunately, the study did not clear up the disagreement over quality of care under managed care. The study's findings that Medicare-managed care patients are more likely to enter the hospital in an emergency situation and have shorter lengths of stay is quite alarming. Yet, the researchers could not find a significant difference in in-hospital mortality rate or hospital re-admission rates. It appears that additional studies will be necessary to determine the true impact that managed care has on quality of care for the elderly.

15.2   TRENDS IN MANAGED CARE CONTRACTING AMONG US HOSPITALS

This study was conducted because there was a paucity of formal research regarding US hospitals that possess or lack managed care contracts. This information would be useful to managed care plans that are looking to expand, hospitals contemplating adoption of managed care contracts, and marketers of managed care products sold to hospitals. This article examines differences among three types of US hospitals. These types include early, recent, and noncontractors of managed care. Early contractors are hospitals that had managed care contracts in or before 1990. Recent contractors are those that initiated contracts between 1990 and 1992. Noncontractors did not have a managed care contract as of 1992.

The study was conducted by Dr. Gautam, Dr. Campbell, and Dr. Arrington (1995), all professors at St. Louis University, which used data from the American Hospital Association (AHA) and the Healthcare Investment Analysts (HCIA). The data set consisted of 4,159 hospitals in the AHA.

The study used various factors to explain why hospitals chose to be early, recent, or noncontractors. These included location, geographic region, type of ownership, multi-institutional affiliation, size, financial and operating performance, reimbursement, and continuum of care. Descriptive statistics were calculated and tests were conducted to identify significant statistical differences between early, recent, and noncontractors. Then logistic regression analysis was performed to identify factors predicting the probability of being an early, recent, or noncontractor. This statistical procedure can calculate the probability that a hospital with that characteristic will be an early, recent, or noncontractor.

Numerous trends resulted from the study, which focused mainly on the differences between early and recent contractors and between recent and noncontractors. First, urban and metro (population of at least 1 million) hospitals formed the highest percentage of early contractors. Early contractors were also typically members of systems or alliances. Early contractors appeared to be those that were financially stable and offered a wider range of services. The ranking showed these characteristics were mainly for early contractors followed by recent and then noncontractors. The numbers also suggest that recent and noncontractors had much in common while early contractors appeared quite different.

Further evidence showed that both recent and noncontractors are predominately rural, smaller in size, have lower case mix, and are financially weaker. Administrators and board members contemplating managed care contracting needed to consider leadership, vision, and risks in their decision making process. Logistic regression was performed for recent and noncontractors. The greatest odds for being a recent contractor included for-profit organizations located in the West North Central and South and Mid-Atlantic states. The organizations most likely to remain a noncontractor of managed care plans were those hospitals in the mountain region and those that included an academic medical center.

The message of this study was that new entrants (during the 1990s) differed significantly from those of the 1980s and contracting with them required new approaches. The first strategy for noncontractors should be to concentrate on forming managed care networks in rural areas since rural hospitals usually lack an adequate number of patients and physicians. They will also be able to handle high resource-demanding patients more efficiently. On the other hand, for-profit hospitals typically form regional networks with multi-sites. They have a reputation for eliminating beds and closing facilities whenever necessary.

In order to continue the study, hospitals in each stage—early, recent, and noncontractors—could be studied on other issues. Other issues that could be explored more in depth include board governance, physician integration, competition, and consumer awareness. A framework can then be developed to help those in the earlier stages anticipate problems.

15.3 MANAGING CARE, INCENTIVES, AND INFORMATION

There is a paucity of empirical literature about the cost-efficiency of alternative methods of managing the care process within hospitals. Most prior studies have documented a "managed care effect" showing that on average, HMO patients consume fewer resources than others, mainly for three reasons: shorter length of stay, less ancillary resource utilization, and fewer hospitalizations. Hardly any literature documents the effectiveness of hospital-based processes such as service line management or actual utilization of resources. This study presents agency theory as a comprehensive theoretical framework for conceptualizing and measuring the hospital's strategy for managing care. It then models the simultaneous impacts on hospital costs of the multiple dimensions that represent the hospital's strategy for managing care.

The investigators (Conrad, Wickizer, Maynard, Klastorin, Lessler, Ross, Soderstrom, Sullivan, Alexander, & Travis, 1996) were associated with the University of Washington (Seattle, Washington) in the departments of Health Services, Cardiology, Management Science, Accounting, Pharmacy, Health Services Organization and Policy, and Economics. They studied the managed care strategies, AHA Annual Survey data, and discharge data of thirty-seven health systems in the Pacific, Rocky Mountain, and Southwest regions of the US. Their intent was to estimate how specific structures, incentives, and processes embodied in the management of care within the hospital ("managedness"), as well as external market factors, actually influence hospital resource consumption.

From within seven health systems, thirty-seven member hospitals were chosen to participate in the study. Each of the sample hospitals could provide complete data for analysis for the years 1991 and 1992. Hospitals averaged 162 staffed beds, comparable to the US average of 173 beds for community hospitals. Hospitals were drawn from Arizona, Colorado, Idaho, Oregon, Utah, Washington, and Wyoming, primarily representing community hospitals rather than academic medical centers. Original hospital surveys and uniform hospital discharge abstract systems were used to characterize the individual hospitalizations according to morbidities and costs. The original surveys supplied data on managed care variables relating to hospital payment incentives, coordination and organization of care delivery, information exchange, and hospital-physician integration. AHA Annual Survey data provided characteristics such as staffed beds, teaching activity, scope of services, and continuum of care. The Bureau of Health Professions file supplied information on total active physicians and specialists per capita by county; InterStudy Competitive Edge data measured the number of HMO enrollees per plan area. Hospitals provided discharge data for the two years for acute myocardial infarction, congestive heart failure, chronic obstructive pulmonary disease, pneumonia, hip replacement, and for the independent variables included in the analyses.

Ordinary least squares regression (OLS) was used with cost per hospital stay (total billed institutional charges per discharge times hospital's overall ratio of cost-to-charges) as the outcome variable. OLS regression equations were estimated for the dependent variable (DV) of cost per discharge. The DV was transformed to its natural logarithm ("ln cost") to reduce skewness and to produce more well-behaved and easily interpreted estimates. Regressions were calculated two ways: (1) including all observations, and (2) excluding outliers (3 standard deviations from the mean). Four categories of independent variables (IV) were used: hospital- and patient-level control variables, managed care variables, market area and regional factors, and hospital-system specific indicator variables to reflect fixed effects of the systems.

Although not definitive (due in part to the non-randomized and small sample size, restricted time periods studied, and the non-specificity of hospital management process models), the study offers some preliminary findings on how to promote hospital efficiencies consisting of:

1. developing payment arrangements under which the hospital assumes economic risk (e.g., capitation),
2. intensifying management of care processes for specific health problems (e.g., care paths), and
3. providing systematic information to physicians on resource consumption in the care of their patients).

Unlike other studies, this one did not find that peer reports to physicians had any significant effect on utilization of resources. Whereas coordination of care delivery lowered costs by 7-12%, product line management raised costs by 8-14%. Hospital-physician integration outcomes indicated that more hospital-employed physicians is related to lower costs, whereas more specialists and exclusive contracts with physicians raised costs 6-12%.

There are a number of business implications found in this study. The patterns of "managedness" and market area characteristics found to be significant could guide hospital administrators who seek to increase efficiencies within integrated delivery and financing systems. While care paths and clinical guidelines were positively related to lower cost and lower resource utilization, product line management was associated with increased costs. Administrative support to facilitate clinical integration should be looked at critically given the negative outcomes of product line management in this study. Energies should perhaps be placed more at the patient care delivery level than at the broader system level. As hospitals merge and look again to physician-driven systems reminiscent of the earlier part of the 20th century, business managers should remain vigilant of the cost implications of physician/hospital contractual arrangements as shown in this study. Where clinical outcomes supersede cost outcomes, the wise manager will know this from the outset and not find him/herself questioning higher costs associated with management practices.

As with most studies, the outcomes of this one are not final and lack the generalization possible from a larger and more geographically representative sample. Also, since an effort was made to under-represent medical centers where costs are known to be higher and resource utilization less efficient because of both the higher acuity levels of patients and the vagaries of medical education, the study is less helpful to such centers that are looking for remedies to higher costs. Business managers should keep a keen eye for where and how the three key variables could be used in any system, however, and monitor the outcome of any of these that are set in place. Also, not to be overlooked in this study is the Agency Theory framework utilized to define "managedness" and to give structure to a review of characteristics likely to have impact on costs and resource utilization. It is at least a beginning place for business managers as they consider the influence of managed care, contracts, and even mergers of smaller systems for economies of scale and scope.

15.4   BUSINESS STRATEGIES PROMOTE COST-EFFECTIVE PATIENT BEHAVIORAL CHANGES

Health Maintenance Organizations (HMOs) are built on the premise that management of health costs versus fee for service (FFS) can reduce overall usage and promote savings to patients and employers (while providing better quality care). To induce these savings, the "gatekeeper" models provide financial incentives/penalties for physicians and patients alike. In most group practices full capitation has not yet reached all markets and groups care for both HMO and FFS patients.

Researchers, Flood, Fremont, Jin, Bott, Ding, and Parker (1998) used patient record data (encounter records, demographic files, clinical records) from a large group practice treating both HMO and FFS patients. The data covered 3.5 years and included 100,000 episodes of treatment for patients under 65. They examined how a group practice (220 providers representing 30 specialties in multiple branch locations) used organizational strategies rather than provider-level incentives to achieve HMO savings. Standard clinic charges were used and then adjusted during payment. They used 1.5 million encounter records providing identical information for services based on CPT-4 codes, associated clinic charge, service provider, HMO-assigned physician (if any), and up to 12 diagnostic codes for office-based services. Medicare patients were excluded due to the benefit structure and payment schedule; Medicaid patients were not in HMOs at the time of the study.

The researchers compared resource utilization of both the FFS and HMO patients. By analyzing data and comparing this to organizational changes, they attempted to find if HMO incentives controlled patient and practice behavior fluctuations. Organizational strategies that encourage desirable behavior among HMO patients and providers will result in lower resource utilization of services and in greater use of generalists for HMO patients. In order to control for disease and case mix, the lower total resources for HMO episodes are largely explained by the provider's specialty (which reflects organizational strategies rather than provider-level incentives).

Earlier studies have focused on the success of HMOs to save money by basing their assumption on the financial incentives that providers react to. They further proposed that providers use least costly resources for HMO patients and the more profitable resources for FFS patients. The research showed that patient and provider behavior responded to organizational strategies designed to work in an HMO environment. Financial incentives played no role in patient choice or the referral patterns of providers. HMO patients used mid-level providers more often and relied less on emergency room or specialist care.

Financial incentives aimed at HMO-patients included co-pays. HMO-patients were encouraged to see generalists in 3 ways:

1. selecting a gatekeeper from a pool of clinic physicians (excluded subspecialties),
2. new enrollees found that generalists—particularly family practitioners—were readily available to accept new patients, and
3. patients preferred to be treated at branch clinics where most generalists practiced.

Organizational changes included marking charts of HMO patients, educational appeals to practice cost-effective care, monitoring and feedback, and exception management.

Regression data indicated a strong trend that patients with poorer health received more resources regardless of insurance. The overall effect of having HMO insurance resulted in the patient receiving significantly fewer outpatient resources. Three important findings were reported:

1. HMO influenced patient and provider behavior by using patient-oriented and physician-oriented strategies to reduce care,
2. HMO care (for the 7 diseases) used fewer expenditures, and
3. HMO insurance did not reduce case mix-adjusted expenditures.

The study confirms that managed care can achieve savings but the savings do not have to apply to those in an HMO only. FFS patients can also be included. Savings occur when patient and provider behavior patterns are adjusted to become more cost effective. The role of organizational strategies in these changes cannot be minimized. By accepting their role as managers as well as physicians, providers can influence patient choice. Providers can also achieve savings without the interference of HMOs within their practices. Physicians have to access their practice data and patterns and use this to change their habits.

The results suggest that HMOs can achieve significant outpatient savings without requiring each provider to change his or her clinical decisions based on the insurance of the patient. By applying management techniques from management courses, physicians can streamline operations, reduce outstanding collections, increase volume, reduce costs, invest in capital, and provide lower administrative costs to serve the patient. Patients can, through education and behavioral changes, become better users of the health system. The study does have some limitation: it did not include Medicare and Medicaid, and was performed on predominantly white, middle-income patients living in a small urban area.

15.5   WHY DO EMPLOYEES KEEP CHOOSING THE HIGH-PREMIUM HEALTH CARE PLAN?

In 1991 Dannon employees were given a choice to stay with their current health care plan or change to a new plan which was the same as the old plan in every way other than offering a lower premium and less hospital coverage (Sturman, Boudreau, & Corcoran, 1996). Management believed that this new plan better suited employee needs, but only 25 percent of the employees switched to the new lower premium plan. The article reports a collaborative effort between The Dannon Company and Cornell University to identify the patterns of employee choices and the actual costs that employees incurred.

The Human Resource (HR) department at Dannon was attempting to shift from an entitlement to a partnership philosophy. Management intended to implement a new pay-for-performance system including more reliance on bonus pay and gainsharing. The first move in this direction was to offer a new health care option which management thought would better serve employee needs, required greater cost sharing, but offered lower premiums. HR expected that the majority of employees would select the new plan, but less than 25 percent selected the new plan.

The new plan was the same as the old plan in every way except for the following differences. The new plan offered a lower premium than the old plan. The new plan only covered 80 percent of hospital related claims while the old plan covered 100 percent of these claims. The new plan had a $200 deductible while the old plan's deductible was $100. Both plans had a similar out-of-pocket cap, and both plans had similar claims procedures, and offered the same amount of choice among health care providers. In fact, the same company administered the two plans.

The researchers believed that two theories suggest possible choice patterns for employee medical benefits: Expected Utility Maximization (EUM) and Prospect Theory. EUM theory suggests that employees will select the plan that maximizes their "expected utility" (makes them better off). The theory also suggests that people are risk averse and will select the plan which has the highest value on the most important dimensions with the most certainty. People will generally prefer lower cost and less uncertainty. Yet each person has a different risk tolerance and differs on what they consider important, so each person has a different utility function. If EUM theory is correct, the researchers would expect to see employees choosing the plan that minimizes out of pocket costs, since all other aspects of the plans are the same. The other theory the researchers point to is Prospect Theory. Prospect Theory says that people facing risky choices (prospects) will react more to losses than to gains, and that gains and losses are judged relative to a reference point.

The researchers collected data on 340 employees at one of the Dannon plants for 1991 and 1992. A total of 287 cases were obtained in both years. The researchers used the data to measure the Out-of-Pocket Cost (OPC) of each employee in the sample. The OPC included premium paid, individual medical charges, and reimbursement characteristics of the selected plan. The researchers then used OPC to measure Financial Regret, which measures the financial consequences for making a non-cost-optimal choice. The researchers tabulated the data and computed the Average OPC and Average Financial Regret for each of the two plans each year. They also calculated the standard deviations of these measurements.

The results indicated that providing employees with a choice of health care plans allowed them to select lower-cost plans. The choice actually saved employees money over the two-year period, an average of $14,236 per year as a group. Providing a choice instead of forcing employees into the new plan actually saved about $36,699 per year. Regression analysis showed that being male, having more children, and higher potential financial regret positively impacted the selection of the plan, which provided the minimum OPC. The results also indicated that women were more likely to choose the high-coverage, high premium plan than men. The low cost decision was even more favorable in 1992 but this may be the result of either employees learning to choose the plan that best meets their needs or employees adapting their spending and behavior to the plan they chose. Overall the results supported the notion that employees' choices differ when changing the reference point and that employees generally choose the low-cost plan when the risk gets higher. These findings support the initial hypothesis formulated by using Prospect Theory.

This study shows that when managers are considering offering a choice of plans to employees the more accurate prior knowledge they have about enrollment patterns the more accurately managers can forecast cost. They will also be able to better educate employees about plan choices, and determine if a choice of plans is of any value at all. In fact the study lends some support to the idea of offering a choice even if most employees will not choose the low-cost choice. Future research might focus on the role of OPC when combined with other plan characteristics such as freedom of choice and the delivery system. In addition future research could collect data on both actual medical expenses as well as employees' predictions about their expenses. Finally future research could be done to determine if employees who did in fact chose the option, which turned out to be low cost, are satisfied that this was the best choice for them.

15.6   MANAGED COMPETITION IN PRACTICE: "VALUE PURCHASING" BY FOURTEEN EMPLOYERS

Managed care now dominates health care delivery in the US. What are the purchasing practices of large companies in the context of health insurance benefits? Little has been published regarding how and why large companies have spearheaded a massive shift in purchasing practices by implementing managed competition. In this study, published in the May/June 1998 issue of *Health Affairs*, the authors examined the activities of fourteen large US companies which have transformed their purchasing of health care benefits. The authors are: James Maxwell, of John Snow, Inc. (JSI) Research and Training Institute in Boston; Forrest Briscoe of JSI and MIT; Stephen Davidson of JSI and the Boston University of School of Management; Lisa Eisen of the University of Bath in England; Mark Robbins of Harvard Pilgrim Health Care and JSI; Peter Temin of MIT; and, Cheryl Young of Mathematica Policy Research in Cambridge, Massachusetts, and formerly of JSI (1998).

The companies studied included Disney, GTE, and American Express, as well as Orange County Public Schools in Orlando and Fireman's Fund Insurance in northern California, among others. The companies were selected for their reputation as innovative health care purchases. The traditional purchasing system handled health care benefits separately from other purchasing activities and was seen as a function of the human resource department. In contrast, by combining principles of managed

competition with other business tactics, these innovative companies created a system of "value purchasing," a hybrid of the private sector's own
design. Value purchasing systems involved organizational change at three
levels:

1. new organizational arrangements,
2. financial incentives for employees, and
3. the formation of a new relationship with health plans through the
   evaluation and monitoring of quality through procurement strategies such as competitive bidding and direct contracting.

New Organizational Arrangements

Structures revolving around financial and managerial skills were implemented within the companies studied. In some companies, this involved
finance executives assuming responsibility for managing health care programs, while in other cases, finance and accounting worked in teams with
human resources. While some of the human resource departments were
skilled in finance, other firms outsourced. Firms often created new organizational structures with which to interface with health care vendors.

Financial Incentives for Employees

Financial incentives, the most widely used component of value purchasing, encourages plans to compete for enrollees by cutting prices or improving quality for the same services. The company sets its premium
contributions according to a "least-cost" plan which meets the company's
minimum standards, then employees bear the cost exceeding this. Thus,
employees are encouraged to assume more responsibility by choosing a
health plan, depending on needs and cost and quality differences. The
majority of the companies have shifted significant premium costs to the
employees, but at different rates and to varying degrees. While the Fireman's Fund, for example moved quickly into managed care and realized
premium savings thereafter, other companies did not adopt the least-cost
strategy. Some companies believed that if employees assumed a portion of
their premiums, they would have adequate incentive to shift into managed
care.

Procurement Strategies and Quality

Some of the companies in the study have given information to employees concerning health care plan quality and satisfaction. Benefits managers

in the study adopted one or more purchasing techniques, most commonly competitive bidding. Just-in-time purchasing and total quality management principles have been used in selection of health plans. One company, Digital Equipment, required managed care plans to develop standards for their own suppliers of health care, thus encouraging improvements in the supply chain. Only a few of the companies have worked with health plans to produce information to support quality analysis. Some of the companies have developed their own standards for quality, including benchmarking, in plan selection. A few of the companies, such as American Express, 3M, and General Mills have cut costs through direct contracting of services with provider groups via participation in a purchasing coalition.

Significant cost savings have been realized from the rapid migration of employees into managed care. However, confidential focus groups at major corporations reflect employee skepticism about the quality of managed care plans. Advantages for employees in the form of lower health inflation and higher quality care may take time to materialize.

REFERENCES

Conrad, D., Wickizer, T., Maynard, C., Klastorin, T., Lessler, D., Ross, A., Soderstrom, N., Sullivan, S., Alexander, J. & Travis, K. (1996). Managing care, incentives, and information: An exploratory look inside the 'black box' of hospital efficiency. *Health Services Research, 31*(3), 235-260.

Flood, A., Freemont, A., Jin, K., Bott, D. M., Ding, J., & Parker, Jr., R. (1998). How do HMOs achieve savings? The effectiveness of one organization's strategies. *Health Services Research, 33*(1), 79-99.

Gautam, K., Campbell, C., & Arrington, B. (1995). Trends in managed care contracting among US hospitals. *Journal of Health Care Financing, 22*(2), 62-79.

Maxwell, J., Briscoe, F., Davidson, S., Eisen, L., Robbins, M., Temin, P., & Young, C. (1998). Managed competition in practice: 'Value purchasing' by fourteen employers. *Health Affairs, 17*(3), 216-225.

Ni, H., Nauman, D. J., & Hershberger, R. E. (1998). Managed care and outcomes of hospitalization among elderly patients with congestive heart failure. *Archives of Internal Medicine, 158*(June 8), 1231-1236.

Sturman, M. C., Boudreau, J. W., & Corcoran, R. J. (1996). Why do employees keep choosing the high-premium health care plan? An investigation of the financial consequences and logic of employees health care plan selections. *Human Resource Management, 35*(3), 317-342.

CHAPTER 16

CLINICAL HEALTH RESEARCH ISSUES

This chapter covers clinical health research studies in such areas as complication rates in knee replacement patients, mammography screening guidelines, prenatal care use by high risk women, hypertension guideline implementation, and other health related issues.

The first study describes the relationship between physician specialty and outcome of ischemic stroke patients. The two physician specialty areas studied were neurologists versus non-neurologists. The study is based on a sample of nearly 150 stroke patients over 40 years of age who were hospitalized within 24 hours of the onset of stroke symptoms. Of the 146 patients studied, 88 were admitted to neurology services, and the remaining 58 were admitted to other services. The study found that stroke-in-evolution patients are the most likely to be admitted to neurology services. Also neurologist-managed stroke patients had a more favorable prognosis, and experienced lower stroke-related mortality. Hence the study provides evidence that the neurologist-managed specialty care is more effective than general care for stroke patients.

The second study describes the use of care and subsequent mortality. The researchers examined the relationship of three self-reported measures

Proven Solutions for Improving Health and Lowering Health Care Costs, pages 229–146.
Copyright © 2003 by Information Age Publishing, Inc.
All rights of reproduction in any form reserved.
ISBN: 1-59311-000-6 (paper), 1-59311-001-4 (cloth)

of access utilization and one health outcome: mortality. The three measures of access were:

1. last general medical check-up or examination,
2. having a regular physician, and
3. health problem during past 12 months for which a physician was not contacted.

The results revealed that none of the three access factors had any statistically significant outcome (mortality) effects on men but the opposite was true for women. For women, not getting a check-up was associated with increased mortality. The relationship of women, access to care, and mortality is therefore explained by the availability of a source of care for general use.

The third study explores the impact of hypertension guidelines implementation on blood pressure control and drug use in primary care clinics. The study was based on a sample of over 1,600 patients. The results indicated that there was a statistically and clinically significant improvement in the proportion of hypertensive patients reaching their blood pressure goals after guideline implementation.

The fourth study covers prenatal care use among high-risk women. The study seeks to measure the relationship between behavioral risks and prenatal care utilization by high-risk and low-income women. The study is based on a sample of nearly 26,000 deliveries over an eight-year period. The results showed high levels of inadequate prenatal care with more than 54 percent of African-American women receiving either inadequate care or no care at all and white women being more likely than African-American women to receive adequate-plus care. The study shows that a large proportion of women receiving inadequate or no prenatal care continue to be a problem to the health care community.

The fifth study evaluates the impact of self-management by nurses on patient outcomes. The study was done at Johns Hopkins Hospital and compared patient and hospitalization characteristics of two types of hospital units. The one type focussed on nursing self-management (SM) while the other type was a traditionally managed unit (TM). Four units of each type were evaluated in the study. The results of the study indicated that there was no difference in the quality of care patients received. However, job satisfaction of the nurses was higher on the SM units than on the TM units.

The sixth study explores the effect of adherence to mammography guidelines issued by the National Cancer Institute in 1977. Data for the study was obtained from four sources. The results of the study indicated that 72 percent of the women in the study had the age-appropriate number of mammography examinations. The study also reported that availability of primary care providers, mammography facilities with tracking systems to remind women of periodic screening, and higher vs. lower HMO market share all increase adherence to screening guidelines.

The seventh study describes in-hospital complication rates in knee replacement problems. The study focuses on the effect of hospital knee replacement volume on the immediate post-operative complication rate during the initial hospitalization. The results of the study revealed that complication rates decrease up to 80 operations per year. Between 40 and 80 operations per year the complication rate decreases by 3 percentage points. Also patients in for-profit, orthopedic and other specialty hospitals were more likely to have complications. And patients in teaching hospitals and high occupancy rate hospitals were more likely to have a complication.

The eighth and final study evaluates the ecological analysis of the first generation of community clinical oncology programs. The study consisted of utilizing data obtained from the National Cancer Institute of all of the Community Clinical Oncology Programs (CCOPs) funded from 1983–1988, using only programs that were funded for all three years. The research question asked how the output of CCOPs was related to patient measures, professional support measures, funding measures, and organizational and structural measures. The research results indicate that the funding level, clinical research experience, and staff level are the most important factors of patient enrollment.

This chapter covered a variety of health issues with both sociological, financial, economic, and social implications.

16.1 PHYSICIAN SPECIALTY AND OUTCOME OF ISCHEMIC STROKE PATIENTS

Is specialty managed care in the case of ischemic stroke more effective than non-specialty medical care? The initial treatment and resulting outcome of the first time stroke patients varies in hospitals depending whether the patients are managed by neurologists or by non-neurologists.

Researchers George Divine, Ph.D., Ronnie Horner, Ph.D., David Matchar, M.D. of Duke University, and John Feussner, M.D. of Veterans Affairs Medical Center in North Carolina (1995) studied data from private, university, and Veterans Affairs hospitals and explored the relationships among patient characteristics, disease seriousness, and the specialty expertise of the attending physician on one to six month patient outcomes of ischemic stroke victims.

The study was based on a small sample of 146 patients, over forty years of age, who resided within 100 miles of Durham, North Carolina, who were hospitalized within 24 hours of the onset of stroke symptoms, who had no pre-existing stroke history, and who lacked any medical condition for which death was likely within six months.

Following the initial ischemic stroke, patients were assessed within 24 hours of admission, and again at 5, 30, 90, and 180 days after admission. The assessment included physical function and the capacity to perform activities of daily living of the patients. Patients were considered to be under neurologist care if they were admitted to neurology services in a particular hospital. Patients were considered to be under generalist care if they were admitted to medicine or family medicine hospitals. Admission services reflected the established admission policies of the hospital. Also, patients admitted to care other than neurology, were not restricted from consulting a neurologist.

Of the 146 patients studied, 88 were admitted to neurology services, 58 were admitted to other services. The study presents strong differences in admission characteristics between neurology patients versus non-neurology patients. The study found stroke-in-evolution patients were most likely admitted to neurology services. Neurologist-managed stroke patients had a more favorable prognosis, experienced differences in diagnostic testing, and experienced lower stroke-related mortality.

This study has critical implications, particularly as hospitals are increasingly run as businesses. In assessing whether to provide specialty versus non-specialty services, a hospital must address all of the pros and cons. The study provides evidence that neurology specialty care is more effective than general care. However, other factors such as competition from other hospitals, available hospital space, personnel, funding, etc. must be analyzed.

16.2 GENDER, CARE, AND MORTALITY

Early analyses of access to health care ignored outcomes of care but focused on resource availability and utilization. Inspired by an Institute of Medicine report that linked timely utilization of care with best possible outcomes, the researchers examined the relationship of three self-reported measures of access utilization and one health outcome (mortality). They looked at availability of a source of care, care not received for perceived medical problems (foregone care), and a third (less traditional) care measure of receipt of general care (i.e., a physician visit other than for illness).

Peter Franks, Marthe R. Gold, and Carolyn M. Clancy (1996) used data previously gathered in the National Health and Nutrition Examination Survey Epidemiologic Follow-Up Study (NHEFS). NHEFS followed a cohort of the US population for up to four years. A prior study of this cohort linked lower mortality with availability of health insurance. The current researchers used survival analyses to relate mortality to the three selected measures consisting of, availability of a source of care, care not received for perceived medical problems (foregone care), and receipt of general care other than for illness. The analyses adjusted for baseline age, race, education, income, employment status, self-report of health, leisure exercise, alcohol consumption, obesity, residence, insurance status, and the presence of morbidity on examination.

Of the 5,687 working age adults in the original study, researchers excluded 74 Asian American and Native American subjects and 614 others who had publicly funded insurance because their small sample size precluded reliable analyses. Reported analyses are based on a sample of 4,491 persons (incomplete baseline analyses accounted for the additional exclusions). Data were analyzed using the statistical package named SUDAAN in this study. SUDAAN uses a Taylor series approximation method to compute variance and allows adjustment for the multistage probability sampling strategy. Because the original data had a large variability skewness of the weights, several known risk factors were found to be nonsignificant. In this study, unweighted analyses was used. Variables affecting oversampling (age, gender, income) were controlled by using them as covariates. Dichotomized answers to three questions were used for baseline access:

1. When did you last have a general check-up or examination, not counting exams made during a visit for an illness;
2. Is there a particular doctor you see regularly whom you would go to if something were bothering you?;
3. During the past 12 months have you had a health problem which you would have liked to see a doctor about but did not for some reason?

Potential confounders were dichotomized or treated as multiple dummy variables: age in years, race, education, family income, health insurance status, employment status, rural versus urban residence, morbidity, self-rated health, smoking status, obesity status, leisure exercise, alcohol consumption. Household size was treated as an interval-level variable.

After adjusting for all other baseline characteristics, the proportional hazard survival analyses revealed that for women not getting a check-up at baseline was associated with increased mortality. In addition, younger women with at least 12 years of schooling and with no morbidity at baseline were associated with lower mortality. No other variable was statistically significant for subsequent mortality. For men, none of the access variables was statistically significant for subsequent mortality. Also non-significant were education, insurance, employment, residence, and exercise. Additional analysis revealed that characteristics became nonsignificant when income was entered into the equation. Therefore, getting a check-up was simply a marker for higher income and had no adjusted independent relationship with subsequent survival. Two final analyses were performed to examine a possible overadjustment from the inclusion of baseline health status and self-rated health status. No significant change occurred in the hazard ratios with these adjustments.

The study suggests that the mortality experience of American women (but not of men) who get general check-ups is lower than the mortality experience of those who do not get regular check-ups. The relationship of women, access, and mortality, is therefore explained by use of resources, not simply by the availability of a source of care for general care.

Two implications are suggested by the researchers. First, exploring the relationship between more frequent use of ambulatory services by women and their subsequent lower receipt of highly technological intensive services may result in health care business practices that lead to improved health outcomes for men and women alike. Health care providers can also use these data to identify vulnerable populations who do not obtain check-ups, and target special services toward increasing their access to and use of health care services. Secondly, accurate measurements of effective access to services will be increasingly essential for assessing and responding to the impact of changes in medical delivery systems. Understanding gender differences in utilization of resources, perceived levels of health, and health outcomes is critical to any effort for developing worthwhile measures of access.

Two additional possible implications not mentioned by the researchers seem apparent. Opportunity exists during well check-ups to provide women with information for enhancing their effective use of the health care system for themselves and their families. This might lead to building networks of health teaching programs to be presented during a well-visit, or perhaps loaned out in the form of an instructional video or other medium between appointments. Also, it was noted that although men are more likely to use care for general check-ups than women, they do so not at their own initiation but at the initiation of employers or insurers. This more passive utilization among men compared with women might account for its less significant relationship to mortality among men. This situation might be subject to a turn-around if, during the context of required check-ups, men were instructed about how to enhance their subsequent utilization of health care services.

16.3   GUIDELINES ON BLOOD PRESSURE CONTROL AND DRUG USE

Despite the sophisticated technologic, pharmacologic, and educational advances made in treating hypertension, there has been a decrease in the percentage of patients with acceptable blood pressure control since the early 1990s. Clinical guidelines have been developed by various organizations such as the Joint National Committee on Detection, Evaluation, and

Treatment of High Blood Pressure. Such guidelines offer specific recommendations on drug use, frequency of follow-up care, and target levels of blood pressure. Guidelines can be used as a map to guide care and as a benchmark in assessing improvement. While many clinics use guidelines, little evidence exists as to the efficacy of guideline implementation.

The research described in the February 1999 issue of the *Journal for Quality Improvement* indicates that a guideline based improvement model used in ambulatory clinics which focuses on organizational changes, rather than on physician or patient behavior, has considerable potential for success. Principal researchers of the study included: P. O'Connor of Health Partners Research Foundation, Minneapolis, MN; E. Quiter of the RAND Corporation in Santa Monica, CA; W. Rush of MinnHealth and of Family Health Services in St. Paul, MN; J. Meland of Family Physicians of Northfield, MN; Ryu of the University of Minnesota (1999).

Description of Study

Hypertension treatment guidelines used in the study were developed by the Institute for Clinical Systems Integration. The guidelines were consistent with those developed by the Joint National Committee and focused on improving blood pressure control and encouraging the appropriate use of two classes of antihypertensive agents, the thiazide diuretics and beta-blockers. A quasi-experimental before-and-after study design was used over a two-year period at each of two primary ambulatory care clinics in Minnesota. Clinic A was located in a medium sized town and had four family practice physicians. Clinic B consisted of eight physically separate clinics, three of which were included in the study and were in the St. Paul metropolitan area.

To be included in the study patients had to be 18 years of age or older, have had the diagnosis of hypertension within the year studied, and must have been seen at the clinic within that period. Out of an initial 1,665 patients, 1,613 subjects were included in the analysis. Bivariate analysis for dichotomous variables was done using the chi-square statistic and the t-test was used for continuous dependent variables. Multivariate analysis was done to adjust for the effects of age, gender, clinic, and number of office visits.

Results

There was a statistically and clinically significant improvement in the proportion of hypertensive patients reaching their blood pressure goals after guideline implementation. Roughly 15 percent more patients were under control at post-guideline implementation. Mean systolic blood pressure, mean diastolic blood pressure, and mean arterial pressure all showed a broad, consistent, statistically, and clinically significant improvement over the study period. After controlling for extraneous variables, the post-guideline versus pre-guideline period was strongly related to better blood pressure control. Clinic A had a 68.8 percent increase in controlled hypertensive patients, compared with a 15.2 percent increase at Clinic B. The proportion of those treated with guideline-recommended drugs did not change pre- versus post-guideline within any age, gender, or clinic strata.

Implications for Business

Guideline implementation resulted in a significant increase in office visits and in increased use of telephone care and mailed reminders to patients. Thus, guideline implementation appears to be associated with increased short-term costs of care. However, the mean decrease in blood systolic and diastolic pressures, if sustained, would be expected to lead to a 15-25 percent reduction in stroke and a 10-12 percent reduction in coronary artery disease. Therefore, the short term cost increase may be offset by later savings related to reduced rates of such complications. It is noteworthy that improvement was related to organizational changes rather than to pharmacologic changes. Active outreach to already identified hypertensive patients, increased use of nursing staff, and physician and nursing education about effective hypertensive care all contributed to a system-wide change resulting in improved blood pressure control.

16.4 PRENATAL CARE USE AMONG HIGH RISK WOMEN

There is a large proportion of women who obtain inadequate or no prenatal care in the United States. In order to improve the distribution of care, a better understanding of who is receiving care and the amount of care they are receiving must first be obtained. The current research literature has many limitations on the distribution and effect of prenatal care. Research is needed on ways in which prenatal care is distributed, the amount of care that is needed, and the dependent relationship between prenatal care and outcomes. This study seeks to measure the relationship between behavioral risks and prenatal utilization by high-risk and low-income women. The study measures separate results for African-American and White women.

The researchers, Leslie L. Clarke, Michael K. Miller, Stan L. Albrecht, Barbara Frentzen, and Amelia Cruz (1999) obtained data for this study from a database maintained by the Department of Obstetrics and Gynecology at the University of Florida that includes information on every woman discharged from the obstetrical unit at Shands Hospital between 1986 and the date of the study. This analysis used complete calendar year data from 1987 through 1994. The patients in the study were low-income (95 percent on Medicaid) and high risk. The final sample used was 25,992 deliveries after disallowing 2,804 cases due to insufficient information.

Over 200 variables were tracked in the database on both mother and infant. Five categorical variables were created to indicate the presence of the following medical problems: antepartum problems, hypertension, "late" antepartum or hypertension problems, gynecological disease, and medical/surgical conditions. Another variable measured behavioral risks of the self-reported pregnancy experiences. Reproductive history was also considered. Standard socio-demographic characteristics such as age, marital status, and years of education were included in the study.

The analysis was stratified by race (White versus African-American). To differentiate between women with no prenatal care and those with some but insufficient care, a modified version of the Adequacy of Prenatal Care Utilization index was used. This index uses information on week of entry into prenatal care, number of prenatal visits, gestational age at birth, and sex and birth weight of infant to determine comparison to the American College of Obstetricians and Gynecologists guidelines.

The frequency distribution of prenatal care utilization by type of medical problem and behavioral risk were examined. Multinomial logistic regression models that predicted the receipt of adequate care as compared to other levels of care were used. These models controlled the key socio-demographic and reproductive factors that are known to affect prenatal care utilization and isolated the effect of maternal medical characteristics and behavioral risks on the level of care received.

The majority of the sample was White with African-American women over-represented relative to the distribution of African-American women served by this clinic in the community. Similar distribution across all categories except the following was found: African-American women were less likely to be married, were more likely to have had a premature birth, and were less likely to have had a spontaneous or induced abortion. A majority of the women had one or more medical problems (83.9 percent), with African-American women having more than White women. More than 7 percent of the women reported using alcohol, more than 4 percent reported current drug use, and many reported using tobacco, with tobacco use higher among White women.

The results showed high levels of inadequate prenatal care with more than 54 percent of African-American women receiving either inadequate or no care at all and White women being more likely than African-American women to receive adequate-plus care. Women who entered before four months of pregnancy and women who entered in later months, both received adequate or adequate-plus care, thus indicating that factors other than months of pregnancy affect visit levels. Women with no medical problems were less likely to receive adequate-plus care which suggests a strong relationship between medical problems and care levels. Drug usage among African-American women and smoking among White women were the behavioral risks that were found to increase the odds of receiving inadequate care. The odds of seeking adequate-plus care increased for women who had a prior spontaneous abortion. However, women who had a prior pre-term birth were strongly associated with both adequate-plus and inadequate care. Previous induced abortions were associated with reduced odds of receiving no care for African-American women and inadequate care for White women. Women younger than 17 and unmarried are more likely to receive inadequate care. Among White women, the more educated are more likely to obtain adequate-plus care. There is no similar relationship for African-American women.

The large proportion of women receiving inadequate or no prenatal care, for whatever reason, continues to be a problem to the health-care community. Some women obtain more care than is necessary while others receive no care. Greater physician involvement and improvements in health-care coverage of prenatal services will increase early entry into care and more evenly distribute care so that a greater number of low-income women will benefit. To more evenly distribute the care, there must be transfers in the amount received by women with no critical risks to those who currently receive inadequate or no care at all. But, if the redistribution of care does not improve the maternal and infant outcomes, then other devices must be sought.

16.5   THE IMPACT OF SELF-MANAGEMENT BY NURSES ON PATIENT OUTCOMES

A major source of concern in the Health Care Industry has been the shortages of registered nurses (RNs) to meet patient care demand, in addition to problems in nurse retention due to dissatisfaction with working conditions. Concern was also expressed that the shortage of RNs could have adverse effects on the quality of patient care. Would a management strategy designed to attract and retain nurses in a hospital affect the quality of patient care? Research has shown that self-managed nursing units have higher levels of nurses' work satisfaction and retention but have no impact on patient post-discharge outcomes.

There were two theoretical bases for the hypothesis. It stated that providing nurses with an opportunity to participate in self-managed units would increase their satisfaction and improve their effectiveness. A hypothesis from this statement was derived saying that the quality of care provided to patients will improve when delivered by nurses that have become highly motivated as a result of being involved with a self-managed unit. The second theoretical basis was derived from a utility maximization view of human behavior that said that nurses in self-managed units would be expected to maximize their financial opportunities and working conditions. A hypothesis based on this view states that the quality of patient care could suffer if nurses were exposed to bad working conditions like long hours etc., and a lack of financial opportunities available to them.

To test these hypotheses, Cassard, Weisman, Gordon, and Wong (1994) conducted research on a unit-based professional practice model (PPM) based on nursing self-management that was designed in 1981 at The Johns Hopkins Hospital (JHH) and was compared on several outcomes against a traditionally managed unit (TM). Patients from PPM and TM units were compared on a number of patient and hospitalization characteristics. The data was collected from patients discharged from eight nursing units in three clinical areas in one hospital. Four of the units were self-managed units and the other four were traditionally managed units. The data was based on six dependent variables:

1. perceived health status,
2. perceived functional status,
3. needs for care,
4. unmet needs for care,
5. unplanned health care visits, and
6. re-admissions to the hospital within 31 days of discharge.

In addition to the six dependent variables, there were six independent variables factored into the study:

1. Type of Nursing Unit,
2. Socio-demographic Variables,
3. Principal Diagnosis,
4. Severity of Illness, and
5. Operative Status and,
6. Nursing Unit length of stay.

There were two main methods of collecting data: patients were interviewed via telephone about two weeks after discharge, and the second source was data from hospital records.

The study produced several statistically significant findings on the variables studied and on their effect on patient outcome. However, the findings did not support or revoke hypotheses comparing the patients from the PPM units versus the ones from the TM units because the independent variables heavily influenced and almost dictated the results of dependent variables. For example, in many cases there were no differences found between PPM and TM patients on measures of perceived health, functional status or additional health care utilization, PPM units had no significant effect on any category of need. However, these results were heavily skewed because of several socio-demographic characteristics that emerged as significant predictors of treatment related to daily activity needs. Women were found to be three times more prevalent in the unmet activity need category because of the nature of their gender and role in life, regardless of being a PPM or TM patient. Also, Length of Stay (LOS) was a significant variable that influenced higher LOS patients to be more prevalent in the unmet activity need category which basically was a result of the seriousness of their reason for hospitalization.

Overall, this analysis showed that unit-based self-managed nursing units in a hospital have no significant effect on patient outcomes. These units do have an effect on the work satisfaction and retention of nurses in a hospital; however, neither of the hypotheses in this case were supported by this study. The findings suggested that the two hypotheses on the effects of self-managed units on patient outcomes cited in the case were offset by each other and therefore produced no effect. This study could be taken a step further using a theory trimming strategy, eliminating the socio-demographic variables to test the effects of the PPM units versus TM units without the effects of independent variables that could influence the outcome of the dependent variables.

Implications of this study are critical for the Health Care Industry in terms of the satisfaction and retention of RNs in hospitals. It showed that if nurses were provided with better working conditions and possibly financial opportunities, there would be a positive effect on their work performance and it would reduce turnover in the industry. There were no significant implications on the effects of self-managed units versus traditionally managed units' effect on patient outcomes based on this study. However, this study provided evidence that socio-demographic variables, especially gender, have a big influence on patient needs and patient outcomes, which is valuable information for improving patient outcomes in hospitals.

16.6   EFFECTS OF MAMMOGRAPHY SCREENING GUIDELINES

In 1977 the National Cancer Institute issued guidelines for mammography screening. Breast cancer mortality is decreased with regular screening mammography. What factors are associated with women's adherence to screening guidelines?

Researchers Kathryn Phillips, Ph.D. from the University of California at San Francisco, Karla Kerlikowski, M.D. from the Department of Veterans

Affairs, Laurence Baker, Ph.D. from Stanford University and associates (1998) measured adherence to NCI guidelines by looking at whether or not a woman had the age-appropriate number of mammography examinations.

Data was combined from four sources: individual level data on women's characteristics and mammography utilization, county-level mammography facilities data, county-level HMO market share data and county-level data on primary care shortage areas. Sequential, multi-part models, where each equation is a subset of the prior equation, were used.

Dependent variables examined were:

1. Ever had mammography
2. Mammography within the past two years
3. Age-appropriate mammography according to NCI guidelines

For the independent variables a "behavioral" model was used including the individual characteristics:

1. Predisposing-age, race, education, family size
2. Enabling-income, insurance, HMO, recent Pap smear, who made the decision for screening
3. Breast problems

Environmental characteristics included:

1. Primary care shortage area
2. HMO market
3. Reminder systems
4. Screening charges

Statistical tests included Chi-square, logistic regression for multivariate analysis, and Hosmer-Lemeshow goodness of fit.

Results included that only 27 percent of the women in the study had the age-appropriate number of mammography examinations. In comparison 59 percent of the women had mammography in the past two years and 70 percent had mammography in the past.

Significant differences across the mutually exclusive groups were found in terms of age, race, education, household size, recency of Pap smear, perception of the decision-making process, breast problems, primary care shortages, and HMO market share.

The fact that only one quarter of the women report adhering to screening guidelines has important implications on practitioners, mammography programs and policies. The finding that a women's report that she participated in the decision to be screened was associated with adherence to a new and important finding. It is a highly significant predictor of adherent versus non-adherent behavior and can be modified in clinical practice.

Environmental characteristics are associated with adherence. Availability of primary care providers, mammography facilities with tracking systems to remind women of periodic screening and increased HMO market share all increase adherence to screening guidelines. These must all be considered when developing new services for women.

16.7   VOLUME EFFECTS ON COMPLICATION RATE IN KNEE REPLACEMENTS

Researchers conducting this study were Edward Norton, Ph.D. from the University of North Carolina, Steven Garfinkel, Ph.D. from the Research Triangle Institute, Lisa McQuay from Glaxo Welcome, David Heck, M.D., from Indiana University, and others (1998) under a research grant from the U.S. Agency for Health Care Policy and Research.

The number of total knee replacements in 1990 was almost double those performed in 1985. The large number of knee replacements leads to the question of what factors influence a good outcome. Total knee replacement outcomes research has focused on outcomes defined as improvements of function, pain relief, prosthesis failure, and mortality. Studies have found knee replacements to be effective. This study focuses on the effect of hospital knee replacement volume on the immediate post-operative complication rate during the initial hospitalization. If hospitals with higher volume have lower in-hospital complication rates, then there is a policy tradeoff between making total knee replacements available at more hospitals to improve access or making total knee replacements available at fewer hospitals to improve the quality of care.

Data from the Health Care Finance Administration Medical Provider Analysis in Review (MEDPAR) was used for the study. These files contain data on 100% of Medicare reimbursed hospitalizations. Medicare Part A was searched for in-patient claims from 1985 to 1990 to identify all hospitalizations in which patients underwent a primary total knee replacement by using the appropriate ICD-9 codes. Exclusions were patients enrolled in HMOs, those whose health status was presumed different from that of other Medicare recipients, patients who reside outside of the United States and several outliers. The final population was 295,473 observations. The dependent variable of interest is an indicator of whether or not the patient had an in-hospital complication. Claims data was used to identify diagnoses that were likely to indicate a complication, including mortality. A group of physicians divided the most common complications into likely, possible, or due to anemia. The most common complication is anemia and this was analyzed separately.

Exploratory variables were divided into hospital characteristics and patient characteristics.

1. Type of hospital—profit, non-profit, government, orthopedic, other specialty, teaching, or member of multi-hospital system.
2. Clientele—percentage of hospital in-patient days for Medicare patients and the occupancy rate.
3. Services offered—presence of physical therapy and presence of out-patient rehabilitation services.

A Logit statistical model for each complication: likely, possible, and anemia was used. A positive coefficient indicated that an increase in the corresponding covariate would increase the probability that a patient had a complication.

The results showed that the marginal effect of volume was nonlinear between 40 and 80 operations per year and close to zero below 40 and above 80 operations per year. This implies that an increase in the number of operations from 40 to 80 per year would decrease the probability of a likely complication by 3 percentage points.

The same is true for the probability of a possible complication. For anemia it is slightly different, the coefficient on volume between 20 and 40 operations per year was negative and highly statistically significant.

Hospital characteristics that were significant were:

1. Patients in for-profit, orthopedic, and other specialty hospitals were more likely to have all complications.
2. Patients in teaching hospitals or hospitals with high occupancy rates were more likely to have a likely or possible complication but less likely to have anemia.

The other characteristics, presence of physical therapy, and out-patient rehabilitation services, were not statistically significant.

A strong time trend in the summary statistics persisted. Each year the probability of a complication rose significantly. The annual increase in the probability of each type of complication was almost constant. A set of regressions showed that there was no difference between 1985 and the other years in the volume and complication relationship.

Noteworthy findings for business:

*   Confirmed the existence of volume outcomes relationships for total knee replacements.
*   Patients at hospitals that do more operations have better outcomes than patients at hospitals that do fewer; specific threshold levels benefit begins at 40 operations per year and is no more once 80 operations per year are performed.
*   Complication rates increase consistently over time along with the number of total knee replacements.

- After controlling for co-morbidities for-profit hospitals have a higher complication rate than other hospitals.

Rather than uncontrolled expansion of knee surgery to increasingly smaller hospitals, decentralization to regional centers where at least 50 and preferably 100 operations per year are assured appears to be the optimal policy to reduce in-hospital complications.

16.8 ANALYSIS OF COMMUNITY CLINICAL ONCOLOGY PROGRAMS

In the area of health services, collaboration has become a necessity in order to survive in today's environment. In a time when the public demands more and more services and expects to pay less is in direct contrast to an industry in which health service activities have become more complex and expensive. However, there is only so much money to go around for funding. With more and more companies in the health services industry teaming up with each other, coordinating activities and allocating funds can pose problems. Such problems are competition for funds, crossing over company boundaries, unequal power to divert funds in one company's direction, levels of investment, problems with coordination, and conflicting interests between companies. Such struggles can result in less productivity and improper use of resources. In order to combat this problem, a framework must be implemented in which factors must be considered when allocating funds to promote adequate performance between the companies, as well as a support system needed to regulate such decisions.

In the April 1993 issue of *Health Services Research,* Janice Schopler published a paper that tried to come up with such a framework by doing an ecological analysis. She decided to use the data collected from the first generation of Community Clinical Oncology Programs (CCOP), which was a nation-wide interorganizational program funded by the National Cancer Institute (NCI) from 1983-1986. This data was chosen because the study of interorganizational relationships suggested that both the organizational and environmental perspectives were necessary to understand why interorganizational relationships meet with varied success. Once the data was chosen, an open systems model was implemented in which inputs from the environment (such as resources, requirements, and political environment), inputs from member organizations (such as size and technology) and boundary spanning structures (form, adaptability) were all-important factors to the output (productivity) of a particular CCOP. The hypothesis that was being tested in this study was whether variation in outputs among the CCOPs was significantly associated with differing levels of environmental inputs, organizational inputs, and measures of structure. The results of the test would be used to identify factors that were important to the development and outcomes of the first generation of the CCOP.

The study consisted of utilizing data obtained from the National Cancer Institute of all of the CCOPs funded from 1983-1986, using only programs that were funded for all three years. When measuring variables, the major measure of productivity of the program's output was the number of patients enrolled on approved research programs for each year. Environmental inputs included measures of population density, organizational dominance, professional support, and NCI funding. These inputs are indicators of potential patients, the potential competition, professional involvement, and the annual dollar amount the NCI provides for direct costs. Organizational variables included measures describing the inputs from member organizations and the structure of the CCOPs. This membership was measured in terms of the number of hospitals, the number of physicians, and the number of support staff. A structural measure was used for the number of position categories, as well as an administrative concentration of these categories. A low ratio indicates a more concentrated administration.

The research question asked how the output of CCOPs was related to patient measures, professional support measures, funding measures, and organizational and structural measures.

After gathering all the data and applying the numbers, a number of observations could be summarized. The first observation was that a majority of variations in outputs between programs could be explained by either the amount of NCI funding, the number of support staff, and the level of clinical research experience. Out of these three, clinical research experience was the most important in the first year. After the program has been established, external funding plays a bigger role in getting patients. The size of the support staff tends to be more of a predictor of an upcoming change in enrollment than enrollment at present. The other variables in the equation such as organizational dominance, professional support, and physicians have a positive influence on outcomes, while the structural area of specialization tends to have a negative relationship. This could be due to a lack of proper interorganizational channels that are needed for these programs to run effectively. When making decisions on what program gets how much money, the proper support staff and technology must be in place for the program to work.

In conclusion, the research results from the data suggest that the funding level, clinical research experience, and the number of staff are the most important factors of patient enrollment. The amount of research experience has a positive correlation with patient enrollment and a negative correlation with changes in enrollment. Another important finding is that certain variables are more important at the beginning of these programs, and in order to expand these programs, different variables must be addressed to succeed.

The implication that this study has for business is that the data collected gives a good example of the way external factors as well as internal factors influence the outcomes of interorganizational systems that rely on external funds. This is similar to joint ventures which come into being in response to new factors that come into play on both an external and internal level. This type of ecological approach provides a good framework which businesses can use to show how different variables become more important as the project continues from year to year.

REFERENCES

Cassard, S. D., Weisman, C. S., Gordon, D. L., & Wong, R. (1994). The impact of unit-based self-management by nurses on patient outcomes. *Health Services Research, 29*(4), 415-433.

Clarke, L. L., Miller, M. K., Albrecht, S. L., Frentzen, B., & Cruz, A. (1999). The role of medical problems and behavioral risks in explaining patterns of prenatal care use among high-risk women. *Health Services Research, 34*(1), 145-165.

Franks, P., Gold, M. R., & Clancy, C. M. (1996). Use of care and subsequent mortality: The importance of gender. *Health Services Research, 31*(3), 347-364.

Horner, R., Matchar, D. B., Divine, G. W., & and Feussner, J. R. (1995). Relationship between physician specialty and outcome of ischemic stroke patients. *Health Services Research, 30*(2), 275-282.

O'Connor, P. J., Quiter, E. S., Rush, W. A.,Wiest, M., Meland, J. T., & Ryu, S. (1999). Impact of hypertension guideline implementation on blood pressure control and drug use in primary care clinics. *Journal of Quality Improvement, 25*(2), 68-77.

Norton, E. C., Garfinkel, S. A., McQuay, L. J., Heck, D. A., Wright, J. G., Dittus, R., & Lubitz, R. M. (1998). The effects of hospital volume on the in-hospital complication rate in knee replacement patients. *Health Services Research, 33*(5), 1192-1210.

Phillips, K. A.. Kerlikowski, K., Baker, L. C., Chang, S. W., & Brown, M. L. (1998). Factors Associated with Women's Adherence to Mammography Screening Guidelines. *Health Services Research, 33*(1), 29-53.

Schopler, J. H. (1993). Ecological Analysis of the First Generation of Community Clinical Oncology Programs. *Health Services Research, 28*(1), 69-96.